Clinics in Human Lactation

History and Assessment: It's All in the Details

Denise Altman RN, IBCLC, LCCE

D1218586

Clinics in Human Lactation

History and Assessment: It's All in the Details

Denise Altman RN, IBCLC, LCCE

Praeclarus Press, LLC
2504 Sweetgum Lane
Amarillo, Texas 79124 USA
806-367-9950
www.PraeclarusPress.com

DISCLAIMER
The information contained in this publication is advisory only and is not intended to replace sound clinical judgment or individualized patient care. The author disclaims all warranties, whether expressed or implied, including any warranty as the quality, accuracy, safety, or suitability of this information for any particular purpose.

ISBN: 978-1-939807-67-0

TABLE OF CONTENTS

PREFACE

I became a Lactation Consultant because of a 40-year-old ex-heroin addict. In 1992, I took a position as a staff nurse working night shift on an OB/Gyn unit at a busy teaching hospital. At the time, I was also preparing to get married and had no children of my own. I liked the idea of helping women through major transitions in their lives-whether it was the birth of a baby or facing the emotional changes related to hysterectomy. Because this was also the county hospital, patients were from all walks of life - young, old, wealthy, street people, prisoners from the local jail, married, and unmarried. During that time, breastfeeding support where I worked consisted of giving mothers a lot of useless rules and little else; most of us in healthcare didn't know how else to help, even when we wanted to.

One night when the unit was slow, I went to check on one of my patients, a woman who had lost her previous children to foster care because of her addiction. She was currently on methadone, and this was her last baby. She was going to have her tubes tied in the morning. She was nursing her baby and because it was quiet, I sat on the edge of her bed while she finished before taking her vital signs. We began to talk, which turned into a real conversation, then an education session. For whatever reason, she opened up to me about her addiction and what she had lost as a result. She talked about buying drugs and the dangerous situations she had put herself into. She explained what breastfeeding her newborn meant to her now during her recovery from her previous life: using words that were simple and from the street. In her straightforward statements, I could hear terms like "empowering" and "victory," although they were not used by her. She told me her story, embedded within her history.

I can't even remember her name, but she taught me well. It was a turning point for me, and I realized that women deserve more than a statement of support, they need someone with knowledge. If I could gain that knowledge, I could really make a difference.

I believe that listening to mothers teaches us more than we realize. Each mother has a story, and it begins with the basic medical questions that can seem so dry and tedious. If we can just use those boring forms as a starting point and allow her to tell us the rest, we can help her meet her goals and also help ourselves. It becomes a circle.

ACKNOWLEDGMENTS

This monograph would never have been started without the encouragement of two of my professional pals: Jan Ellen Brown and Diana West, both of whom have given me advice, encouragement, and a push whenever I need it. Along the way, I received tremendously valuable input and resources from the Greater Columbia Mothers of Twins Club, Immaculate Body Piercing, staff at Providence Hospital, and my backup Chaka Davis, who is also the nurse expert on very tiny, fragile babies in our community. I never would have completed it without the support of my husband Jim and my three credentials (Jamie, Christina, and Genevieve), who allowed me time off from my real job.

Lastly, of course, this monograph starts and ends with the mothers who trained me, and always, with their stories.

Chapter One

BEFORE BEGINNING

Overview

The two most important elements of providing professional breastfeeding support are taking a complete history and performing a detailed physical assessment. Without these two fundamentals, the development of a breastfeeding plan, or even accurate identification of a problem, is impossible.

In spite of this, taking a history, in particular, can often seem too lengthy a process when understaffed or short on time. In addition, a complete physical assessment, including observation of a full feeding, is often cut short or eliminated because patient volumes are great, or the necessity of a full observation isn't recognized. This can lead to increased problems for the feeding dyad, heavier financial burdens for both the family and the healthcare system, and emotional costs for the mother and baby. When a feeding assessment is cut short, the mother may also feel frustrated because of a perceived lack of assistance or interest by the Lactation Consultant.

Ideally, the initial elements of the history should be completed before the physical assessment begins. Although there is some overlap, the information obtained will offer clues or triggers for close observation or further investigation. In addition, during the assessment, findings different from the norm should be reported to the primary caregiver for further evaluation. During the history and assessment, patient education should be ongoing as needs are identified.

This monograph will cover the important elements of the patient history, along with rationale, as well as steps for physical assessment on a basic level. Variations from the norm will not be explored in great detail because the intention and focus is on the basic process. For consistency throughout this monograph, the breastfeeding advocate will be identified as the Lactation Consultant (LC), although it is understood that readers may be from a variety of practice or volunteer settings. Babies are referred to in gender neutral terms.

Process

Healthcare professions all have their own individual standards for organizing the delivery of care. Most of these are similar to the scientific method, beginning with an identified problem and ending with the tested theory. Perhaps the closest to the role of the LC is the nursing process. Typically stated in general terms, the nursing process can easily be adapted to fit the needs of the mother and baby. The process functions in a flowing format, beginning again after evaluation to determine new needs or to change any element of the process that does not contribute to the desired outcome.

The process for a seasoned LC is often at an unconscious level, and evaluation may be occurring within the steps of the process, rather than after a formal implementation of a plan. However, the theory is still applicable, and the LC relies heavily on critical thinking skills within this type of approach. An example of the Lactation Consultant process that is based on the nursing process is shown in Figure 1.

The approach for initiating the process is always the same, regardless of the patient's level of care. Whether the mother delivers by cesarean section or has a vaginal birth, or the baby is in the NICU or at home; the beginning is

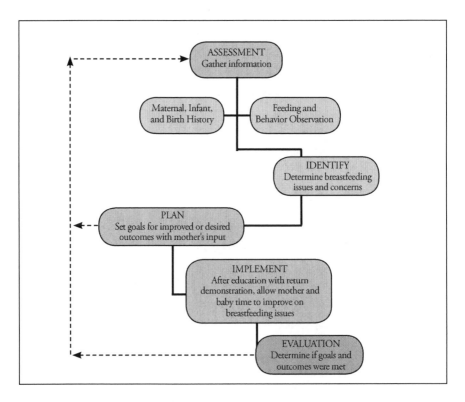

Figure 1: The process of support by the Lactation Consultant

always data collection: first you take the history. Then, you do the maternal and infant physical and feeding assessments.

Because the LC has two individuals functioning within one scope, assessment continues within the plan and implementation phases, demonstrated in Figure 1, with a line back to the start of the process. LCs must be fluid throughout the assessment because data often changes.

Culture, Ethnicity, and Belief Systems

Cultural competence and/or cultural sensitivity have become blanket terms, not only within the healthcare community, but also within business, academic, and almost any other field. As individuals learn to think globally, more become aware of differences in one another. Often, cultural competence is thought to be addressing the needs of the foreign or non-U.S. born individual. However, the reality applies to all individuals, as each one has their own beliefs, languages, behaviors, and/or faith systems. In other words, everyone the LC encounters has their own culture. One literal definition of culture is "the totality of socially transmitted knowledge of values, beliefs, norms, and life ways of a group that guides their thoughts and behaviors" (Potter & Perry, 2005).

Euro-American values are a term that applies to the most commonly held beliefs and characteristics of persons in the United States. This includes: a belief in individualism, a belief in informed consent, orientation toward clock time, and a belief in a faith order of God first, then humans, followed by other living creatures. There are also commonly held values about competition and winning, the right to defend oneself, family or property, a faith in science and technology to improve the human condition, and even that illness in the body, mind, and spirit are separate (Lipton et al., 2002).

This means that how and what the nursing mother is taught is often based on the assumption that the mother and the LC are like-minded. Because the approach may be based on commonly held theories and values, there is a risk that the message may be received incorrectly, devalued, or misunderstood. While the LC cannot possibly be an expert on every type of culture and belief system, there is an expectation that she will have a respect for them, as well as a willingness to explore other cultural characteristics to increase her own knowledge base. Many patients, when questioned about postpartum adjustment, foods, environment of support, and taboos are very willing to share their background with someone genuinely interested in learning and eager to accommodate them.

Faith beliefs should also be addressed, particularly if a patient's faith can potentially impact the breastfeeding experience. Assumptions about a faith may not be valid, for example, not all Jews are kosher.

Example One: A devout Catholic will not practice what she considers to be artificial methods of birth control. Breastfeeding as part of natural family planning is acceptable, so she will need solid educational reinforcement on feeding frequency and duration. She will also need to be questioned and possibly educated during the history about parenting techniques, since some of the more popular programs stress timed feedings, which can increase fertility risks.

Example Two: If the mother is a Jehovah's Witness who refused blood products after a postpartum hemorrhage, she should be further assessed for low supply risk. This can include obtaining her latest blood count results, evaluating her diet for iron rich foods, checking vitamin supplements to make sure they include additional iron, determining frequency and duration of feedings, and assessing intake during the observed feeding. This mother may need to be referred to a dietician to better meet her new health needs, although this is often taught in classes for church members.

> *Teaching Tip: How a mother looks or sounds does not necessarily indicate who she is. Even a mother who is a first or second generation American will have some belief practices that tie to her cultural background. For example, the new mother born and raised in Georgia and speaking with a southern accent may be descended from a mother who emigrated from Korea when she was 20. The new mother, apparently acculturated, may still require warm foods and therapies after delivery. In the Korean culture, anything cold is shunned during pregnancy and the initial postpartum period under the concept of yin and yang. The LC who typically recommends ice packs for engorgement will need to be respectful of this cultural need.*

Cross-Cultural Communication

In many countries, communication of information for decision-making can follow very specific guidelines. In some cultures, the head of the household functions as the spokesperson and needs to be identified, such as the husband in the Puerto Rican family. During conversation, Chinese families will avoid eye contact with a caregiver or authority figure as a sign of respect. They may also feel that asking questions is disrespectful. The LC should be aware of the cultural populations in her community and be familiar with their attitudes, beliefs, and behaviors.

Written and verbal language barriers can be extremely challenging under any circumstances. Sometimes, a family will bring their own interpreter, but if not, the LC may have to identify other resources. Hospitals and other healthcare organizations may keep a list of employees who are fluent in other languages. Generally, nursing supervisors, patient advocates, or directors have access to this information. If there is an organizational intranet, this may also be a resource that is readily available within the system.

Large healthcare organizations typically subscribe to an interpretation telephone system, such as LanguageLine or TeleInterpreters. These companies provide medical interpreters for approximately 150-200 languages, although usage is very expensive at $4/minute. Generally, language lines are used in critical situations or when other options are not available. Other resources may include local interpretation companies or advocacy groups, such as Hispanic Outreach. There are even Internet sites that will translate sentences into a variety of foreign languages without a fee, although this can get unwieldy when a lot of information must be communicated. A tip sheet regarding effective use of an interpreter is attached (Attachment A).

The LC should have written materials in a variety of languages to reinforce common breastfeeding topics discussed during a consultation. Effectiveness of written materials will, of course, depend on the mother's ability to read her own language, which should be assessed as part of the history. This seems basic, but is often forgotten.

Attachment A

TIPS FOR WORKING WITH AN INTERPRETER

1. **Brief the interpreter** – Before beginning the interview, introduce yourself and your client to the interpreter and give the interpreter specific instructions on what needs to be done or obtained.

2. **Speak directly to the client** – Communicate directly with your client, and look at your client during the interview, as if the interpreter were not there. The interpreter will relay the questions you ask to the client and will relay the client's answers back to you.

3. **Speak naturally, not louder** – Your client is not deaf. Talking louder will not help them understand you. Speak at your normal pace. Speak in one or two sentences, enough to convey your thought, then pause to allow the interpreter time to deliver the information to the client. If something is not clear or if you are going too fast, the interpreter may ask you to slow down or clarify.

4. **Ask if the client understands and ask her to repeat instructions back to you** – In some cultures, a person may say yes or nod their head, even if they don't understand, just to be polite. Make sure your client understands by having her repeat instructions and information back to you.

5. **Do not ask the interpreter's opinion** – The interpreter's job is to translate information. He or she should not allow personal opinion to color the interpretation.

6. **Understand that everything you say may be interpreted** – Avoid private conversations during the interview. Whatever the interpreter hears may be interpreted. Avoid interrupting the interpreter while he/she is interpreting.

7. **Avoid using jargon or technical terms** – Neither the client nor the interpreter may know what you are talking about. Be sure to clarify unique vocabulary and provide examples if needed to explain a term.

8. **Understand that it may take longer to conduct the interview** - When working with an interpreter, it may take twice as long to conduct the interview. Many concepts have no equivalent in other languages, so the interpreter may have to describe or paraphrase your questions.

9. **Slow down if reading from text** – People often speak more quickly when reading from written text. Slow down and make sure the interpreter keeps up with you.

10. **Be sensitive to the client's culture** – During the interview, the interpreter may help you find culturally appropriate ways to ask questions that might be offensive to the client. The interpreter is usually more familiar with the culture and customs of the client.

11. **End the interview** – It is up to you to draw the interview to an end, not the interpreter. Be sure to thank the interpreter for their efforts.

Adapted from Language Line Services.

Chapter Two

DOCUMENTATION AND COMMUNICATION

HIPPA regulations state that signed consent must be given before the transfer of personal health information begins. In the hospital or birth center setting, this is already obtained for the LC upon admission. However, outside of these settings, consent must be obtained in written form by the LC at the point of direct contact, before anything else occurs. In the case where professional telephone support is given, verbal consent is obtained and must be well documented.

In order to obtain an accurate and complete history that is clinically relevant, as well as consistent between patients, there must be a documentation tool. The tool can be either software or a paper form (or a combination), and should be specific to lactation, while structured within a format that creates an organized flow.

Electronic Documentation

For the inpatient focused lactation consultant (ILC) in a hospital or birth center, most of the information required on a history form is already within the medical record and does not require duplicate documentation. The ILC will actually be able to spend less time gathering information as a result, but she must be familiar with the chart layout. Most hospital records are now electronic and may be located entirely within a documentation system, such as QS/Centricity, McKesson, or Watchtower (all company as well as system names), until discharge or printed out and placed on the physical chart every 24 hours. Organizational policies regarding hard copies vary widely, along with documentation systems.

Most electronic documentation systems follow a basic software format, but have been personalized to meet organizational needs. Organizational standards for electronic health records (EHR) are overseen by the Healthcare Information and Management Systems Society (Moody et al., 2004). Typically when a large healthcare organization purchases a software system, the manufacturer works with the Information Systems department to personalize a basic template to better meet organizational needs. Representatives from various practice areas may be involved to customize the system to their specific departments. Often, unless the breastfeeding support program is very large or has a visible leader advocate, the EHR does not reflect documentation needs of the LC. Added to the complexity of the documentation is that there are two individuals functioning together (the mother and baby), with each having unique physical, behavioral, and emotional characteristics. This is a significant challenge to overcome in creating a personalized system.

The benefit of the EHR is accessibility and time. A record can be accessed from any terminal within the organization, provided the user has specific permission, usually password and account driven. A record often remains active within the system for approximately 30 days post-discharge. From the patient support standpoint, the LC performing follow up calls, consulting in an outpatient clinic, or visiting the bedside of a readmitting patient can easily review the history and plan of care without having to wait for a paper file from Medical Records or retain records of her own.

Forms

Paper or hard copy documentation can be on a "check box" or "fill in the blank" form that is specific to breastfeeding. There may be a combined form (Attachment B), or the history (Attachment C) and assessment (Attachment D) may be on two separate forms. A lactation-specific form will allow the LC to retrieve only pertinent, critical details, and place them in one location on the medical record, making it easier to identify potential feeding or milk production issues, as well as target areas where additional information is needed. By using or creating a specific document for this purpose, the LC will spend less time taking the actual history. The general flow of the form should include information on demographics, maternal health, pregnancy, birth, infant characteristics, and feedings. There should be adequate space to note additional details or variations from the norm throughout the form. The history form is an effective tool to be used for record reviews and trending, as well (Riordan & Auerbach, 2004).

Teaching Tool: A clear assessment form is an excellent tool for communicating with the primary caregiver, not only to promote and support the advanced practice role of the LC, but also for continuity of care for the patient. The ILC can place a copy of her notes with the progress notes on the physical medical record. The OLC (outpatient LC) or PPLC (private practice LC) can send a fax of her notes with an explanatory cover sheet to the medical office.

Attachment B   Combined H&P Created by Elizabeth Brooks

Elizabeth C. Brooks, JD, IBCLC
International Board Certified Lactation Consultant (LLC EIN 23-3045350)
7906 Pine Road – Wyndmoor, PA 19038 – (215) 836-0591 – Fax (215) 836-0591 – ECBIbclc@yahoo.com – IBCLC Certification: 197-13407

File No.:
Date of Consult

Breastfeeding Assessment

Mom _____

Address _____

Phone _____   Email OK? _____

Ped _____

OB/CNM _____

Birth and lactation history
p _____ g _____ vaginal _____ c/s _____ VBAC _____ induction _____
epidural/none _____ forceps _____ vacuum _____ pitocin _____ epidural _____
If other? _____
fertility/other issues _____
postpartum bleeding _____
meds/medication _____

Breasts _____ soft _____ full _____ firm _____ engorged
surgery/type _____
Mom prems _____ MER _____
pain/other _____
sore/other _____
breast change in pregnancy? _____

Baby _____   M F

DOB _____   Gest age at birth _____   Present age _____
Birth weight _____   Lowest weight _____   current recent wt _____

Baby currently feeds _____ times/day, approx time _____
Urine _____ times/day   Stool _____ times/day, color _____
% Bmilk _____ : _____ % at breast _____ % EBM
% formula _____ mode of supplt _____

Milk transfer at consult _____
Audible swallows _____
Satsf after feeding _____

Baby's weight at consult _____ wt/oz _____
Prenatal: needs each 24 hours in order to gain:
8 feeds/day = _____   10/day = _____   12/day = _____

Oral-digital exam
lip seal YN   hard palate normal   bubble/high
tongue-lower gum line YN   tongue touching YN
tongue-cup/cup YN   ext reflex triggered YN
frenulum thick YN   suction pig-pellet YN
peristaltic tongue YN   other

11

Nipples: flat inverted everted compressible
diameter S M L ___ on length S M L ___ cm
tender painful no pain
nipple shape intact/perfect color pre-feed
post-expression drop/stem
cracked/other

Position taught/observed
cradle
cross-cradle
football
prone
side-lying
standing

Position and Latch
Mom's preferred position
Baby aligned/nose-nipple aligned Y N
mouth opened wide Y N
nose points to nipple Y N
deep or shallow latch
Baby supported done Y N
gloves and stools for support Y N

Technique/
equipment taught
skin-to-skin
breast compression
manual expression
nipple shield use size ___
hospital grade pump
other pump
tube feeding at breast
tube feeding by finger
gavage/other
dropper/other
paced bottle feed
other

Care plan/
instructions provided
APNO
non-latching baby
sore nipples
pre-term baby
delaying engorgement
exclusive MER/increase supply
low supply
slow to gain baby
expected outlet
expected tongue tie
expected thrush
plugged duct/mastitis

L

L

Milk supply (in Day ___)
colostral
low
moderately
moderate/high MER

Notes:

Attachment C

HISTORY ONLY FORM

Mother/Baby History for Lactation Consultation

Demographics

Mother's Name_____Date of Birth _____

Address_____City_____Zip_____

Husband/partner_____Phone(home)_____Cell_____

Email_____Mother's Doctor_____Phone_____

Baby's Name_____BirthDate_____ Sex_____

Baby's Doctor_____Phone_____

Reason for Consult

Breast/nipple pain ___Poor nursing __Slow weight gain ___Supply problem

Other: _____

Who else is helping with problem?_____ How did you hear about

All The Best?_____

Health History

Any medications/vitamins/herbs_____

_____

Medication allergies_____

Food allergies_____

Please check if applicable:

___Smoker ___Infertility ___Postpartum hemorrhage

___Alcohol ___Pregnancy loss ___Thyroid disorder

___Depression ___Anxiety disorder ___Pituitary disorder

___Breast surgery ___Diabetes ___Polycystic ovarian syndrome

___History of any abuse

Other medical conditions_____

Surgical history_____

Other children/age(s):_____

Past breastfeeding experience:_____

Pregnancy History

Breast changes? size__nipple darkening __leaking __tenderness___other__

Prenatal classes attended:_____Where?_____

Complications during pregnancy?_____

Birth Information

Where was the baby born?_____ How many weeks

pregnant?_____

Labor: please check

Spontaneous_____ Pitocin____Cytotec_____ Prostaglandins_____

Membrane stripping_____ Rupture_____

Pain control during labor? Breathing techniques_____ Epidural___

Nubain___

Delivery: Vaginal___   Vacuum___   Forceps___   C/Section

(planned or emergency)___

Time:_____ Complications?_____ Apgars _____

Baby:

Birth wt_____ Discharge wt_____ Most recent wt/date_____

Maturity rating (Ballard score)_____

Any problems after delivery?_____

Time of first breastfeeding?_____ How was it?_____

Was a full feeding assessed by an LC?_____ How many visits?_____

Were there any recommendations?_____

Any supplement?_____ Reason:_____ How was it given?_____

Room in or to nursery?_____

Breastfeeding History

Number of breastfeedings/24hrs____ Avg length_____ How often_____

Longest sleep period (baby)_____ Supplement/how much/how

often_____

How long have you experienced the current problem?_____

Output over 24 hours:

# of BM's_____ Color_____ Amt_____ #wet diapers_____

Most common infant state: _____ Fussy _____ Alert/calm _____ Sleepy

Social/home: _____ Calm _____Busy _____ Help from: _____

Mother's current breastfeeding goals: _____

Comments/other information or details: _____

_____

The above information is complete and correct to the best of my knowledge.

_____(Patient Signature)

Completed by LC:

_____

Attachment D

_____

Assessment Only Form

All the Best **Breastfeeding Assessment (Hx attached to pt file)**

Mother's name_____ Today's date/time_____

Baby's name_____ Age today_____

Reason for consult_____

OB_____Pediatrician_____

Birth weight	D/C weight	Today's weight	Postfeed/ side	Postfeed/ side	Total intake

Breast/Areola	Nipples/Areola
Size/shape	Shape before
Density	Shape after
MER	Color after
Supply	Integrity

Comments _____

_____

Physical Condition of Baby	At Breast Behavior
Appearance	Actions during feed
Skin	Position
Head/posture	Organization
Oral structures	Suck/swallow bursts
Tongue motion/suck	Duration of active feeding
State	Supplement given

Comments _____

_____

Lactation Consult, page two

Name_____

Impression/analysis_____

_____

_____

_____

_____

Plan/techniques _____

_____

_____

_____

_____

Education done (if checked):

___Milk production ___Breast compression ___Signs of adequate intake

___Latch assessment ___Pumping ___Normal infant states ___Positioning

___Milk storage ___Bottle introduction ___Sore nipple care

___S/S infection ___ Burping/comfort for gas ___Hydrogel drgs

___Nutrative/non- nutrative suck

Other:_____

Equipment needed: _____

F/U_____Report to:_____

Signature:_____

Lactation Consultant: _____

Charting Methods

Another option would be written or flow charting. Narrative charting flows like a story, with a beginning and an end. S.O.A.P. charting is a mnemonic that stands for **Subjective** (what the mother states), **Objective** (what is passively seen or observed that supports the subjective information), **Assessment** (in depth visual and physical evaluation of the mother, baby, and the feeding), **Plan** (results of previous information, problem identification, and a plan to work toward resolution of the problem). Both styles of flow charting may require more time for documentation, even when the LC is proficient, but they add more detail and clarity when done correctly. Regardless of the documentation tool, charting is generally done to note by exception or variation from the norm, unless stating what is normal is important to the full assessment, such as observing the mother perform the steps or techniques for proper latch. For example, documentation isn't necessary for a baby that has no observed difficulty with breathing before or during a feeding and is not at risk for respiratory compromise. However, when audible swallows occur during a feeding assessment, this should be noted, even though it is expected. Audible swallows are a part of a full latch assessment and support the presence of milk transfer.

Examples: Case Presentation One is an example of S.O.A.P. charting at a basic level for use in an outpatient or home setting with the focus on assessment. The medical history is separate; the charting example primarily covers the assessment.

Case Presentation Two is straight narrative charting. This was a second visit, follow-up to an outpatient consultation, and contains additional or revised medical history, reassessment, and evaluation.

Both cases are incomplete and are used here as documentation examples only.

Case Presentation One-Home Visit for Intake Assessment - S.O.A.P. Charting

<u>**In Home Consult**</u>   **June 30, 2005/0945**

Patient: Susan Soap (husband/Sam)
123 Charting Road, Columbia, SC 29999
Home: 803/123-5678   Cell: 910/123-4567
OB: Smith (new) 803/789-4561   Ped: Dr. Kidd 803/569-4789
Infant's name: Shelly Soap
DOB: 1/30/05   Current Age: 5 mos
Birth wt: 10lbs, 11 oz
D/C wt: 10lbs, 4 oz (from NICU after 10 days)
Prefeed (today): 18 lbs, 11oz Post feed: 18 lbs, 15 oz   Total Intake: 4 oz

Hx-Contact by pt's husband for home consultation for perceived low milk supply. Pregnancy by in vitro (male related). Pt delivered in North Carolina at term by scheduled c/s for Preeclampsia. Infant to NICU with heart/lung defects repaired by surgery. Pt pumped; infant to breast at 7 days. Fed well EBM/bottle and breast without problems for 5 mos. Pt's husband contacted North Carolina MD who inst him to schedule lactation consult and OB/Gyn f/u as precautionary. Self-referred via ILCA website. Pt taking PNV only. Additional medical history attached.

    S-Pt states infant feeding about q3h with 1 long sleep period x 8hrs. Feeds approx 10-15 min, one breast per feeding. Pt states that she can pump 6-8 oz from other breast, but is now getting 3-4 oz. She states that she can pump 16-20 oz at once first thing in the AM. Pt states reduced output when pumping and feels "a knot" under her left breast. States no fever.

    O-Infant appears healthy, developmentally appropriate. Frequent smiles with hunger cues before feeding. Breasts bilaterally slightly firm, no engorgement. Small nodule palpated at 5 o'clock position below LT breast; appears to be blocked milk duct; no erythema. Pt states that nodule has decreased in size over last 24 hours. Pt wears regular (non-nursing) underwire bra, appears tight fitting-fabric is taut.

    A-Pt initiated feeding in football position. Infant latched immediately, lips flanged outward, tongue over gum, cheeks rounded, accessory muscles visualized; audible swallows. Infant rapid suck pattern, MER almost immediate. Pt does not c/o pain. Fed at RT breast x 10 minutes

19

with intake of 4 oz. Pt states infant takes 4-5 oz by bottle for feed. Appears satisfied, refuses to latch again for additional intake. Pt states this is normal feeding. Infant smiling and cooing after feed x 15 min, then gradually feel asleep.

P-Inst to feed on LT in varied positions for next several feeds to resolve blocked duct. Warm moist heat before feed with massage as well. Avoid wearing a bra while blocked; recommend fitting with local retailer for underwire nursing bra if style is pt preference. Discussed s/s mastitis although none present at this time. Pt using Pump In Style Advance (new) which is not functioning properly, motor is rattling. Inst on process for replacement, pt states husband will f/u. Questions answered about blocked ducts, milk production and supply, diet and exercise, pumping, milk storage. Reinforced f/u with OB/Gyn. Pt verbalized understanding of all. Positive reinforcement given.

Report faxed to Dr. Smith, Dr. Kidd.

Linda Lactation, IBCLC
Business or organization name
803/111-1111

Case Presentation Two - Outpatient Follow-up for Insufficient Supply - Narrative Charting

Outpatient Consultation/Follow-up (2)　　　1/10/08, 1530

Mary Turner/Nick

Contact by Dr. Obstetrician's office. Requesting information regarding Rx's for Ductal Yeast. Information from "Breastfeeding: Diseases and Conditions" sent by fax. Office will call in Rx of Difflucan 100mg x 2 weeks.

Contacted by pt this morning. Feedings and milk supply not improved. Infant has had 1 BM in 24 hrs. Pt is extremely fatigued, states "feedings are taking an hour" and husband is at work. Has support from family for home care but not infant care. Brief consult completed for supplement plan. Husband present for consult.

Breast tissue appears fuller but not firm. Pt used PIS x 20 min on moderate vacuum, high speeds; doesn't have parts for hospital grade pump and wants to continue with PIS. Return of 15 cc EBM. Placed in finger feeder with 15cc Lipil to equal 30cc total. Infant latched onto Lt breast in cradle position, no c/o pain by pt. Feeding tube slipped into infant's mouth. BF x 20-25 minutes, taking all of supplement. Tolerated feeding well. Burped by husband. Inst pt to sleep until 1800 feeding and use support for infant care. Inst to continue to pump x 20 before feeding, latch infant, and use EBM to supplement while feeding; making sure that total volume is 30 cc. Feed q2h with 1 four hour rest during night; min 8 feeds/24hours. If pt needs sleep period tonight, pump, then have husband finger feed EBM with Lipil as needed to equal one ounce; has demonstrated use before. F/U with Ped in AM for wt check and call for feeding plan based on infant assessment. Pt and husband verbalized understanding of all. Will send report to Dr Pediatrician.

Linda Lactation, IBCLC

Business or organization name

803/111-1111

Information Application

The OLC can obtain a copy of the original history form created by the ILC. There should be space for a basic addendum, which is used to obtain details regarding the breastfeeding experience from the mother, covering events after discharge - typically the first week or two of the postpartum period.

For the PPLC, a history form is generally more time consuming and detailed since she can't rely on the hospital medical record. Even though this is a paper form, it is almost a necessity that this tool at least be initiated in an electronic format. To save time, it can be emailed to mothers with Internet and printer access, to be completed before the actual consultation. If this is not an option, it can also be completed over the phone by the PPLC, a trained assistant, or intern; then reviewed by the LC with the mother for clarity, accuracy, and additional information if needed.

When completing a separate assessment form, generally the only elements of the history form that is transferred are names and date of birth. When these forms are combined, the assessment is often completed in a separate location. Even with check boxes, the assessment has space for comments and flow charting because individualization is critical.

The Interview

Information obtained from forms or medical records is somewhat limited, regardless of how detailed the form. After retrieving basic, statistical-style information, the best way to get the most details is from the mother herself. This is accomplished in an interview format. The questions on the form are simply a starting point, a way to identify when further information is needed. Multiple communication techniques and observations are important for accurately and completely collecting data. Information collected from the interview is often greatly subjective, but that does not make it any less valuable.

Brunner and Suddarth have created an excellent list of interview guidelines to obtain an accurate and complete heath history (Smeltzer & Bare, 1992). The following guidelines are generally stated, but follow a specific flow, adaptable to any setting.

1. The interviewer approaches the patient as a unique individual. The interviewer puts the patient at ease and provides for her comfort.
2. The interviewer permits the individual to express herself fully.

3. The interviewer uses a health history form to guide the interview, and adjusts the sequence of questions to coincide with the flow of conversation.

4. The interviewer demonstrates an understanding of the nature and intensity of the patient's problem.

5. The interviewer takes into account the person's cultural background.

6. The interviewer is aware of his or her own feelings and attitudes.

7. The interviewer is attuned to nonverbal communication and learns to recognize gestures that convey defensiveness, hostility, confidence, impatience, and so on.

8. The interviewer communicates in a manner that is consistent with the individual's level of understanding.

9. The interviewer terminates the interview in an appropriate manner that summarizes the information obtained and ensures that the patient has understood major points discussed (Smeltzer & Bare, 1992).

All interviews should begin with the LC introducing herself to the mother and anyone else who will be present for the consultation, sometimes referred to as orientation (Potter & Perry, 2005). The LC should be careful to clarify her role with regard to breastfeeding support for the mother and baby. This is particularly important in the inpatient setting where the mother is often overwhelmed by individuals all wearing similar uniforms, making everyone from Environmental Services to the Anesthesiologist look exactly alike. The LC should also establish a rapport with the mother before attempting to extract personal information or picking up the baby.

Open-Ended Questions

As the patient recounts her experiences, ask open-ended, rather than simple "yes or no" questions. In particular, questions that address the mother's perception are important, since how she feels about a particular situation impacts the actual experience.

Example: "Did the first feeding go well?" will likely give you an accurate answer of yes or no, but you will then have to continue with multiple questions to find out details. Instead "How do you feel the first feeding went?" is a better question because this allows the mother to recall the event, rather than giving a pat answer. She may also take this opportunity to verbalize early frustrations and concerns, which will offer the LC a teaching moment and also provide the mother a sense of relief and the ability to move forward in the learning process.

Active listening, similar to a tool called reflection, is critical when interviewing the mother. This is where the interviewer (LC) has almost a passive role in the process after asking an open-ended question by waiting for the mother's response. The LC should listen to all that is said, giving her full attention to the mother. She should then repeat back what she hears, using her own words to rephrase what the mother has said for clarity. Only after the communicated idea or experience is clear, should the LC write or type the response on the form. If the LC enters the response while the mother is speaking, the message is sent that the form is more important than the mother.

Example: When asked to clarify why the mother said the first breastfeeding was bad…

Mother: *"It was nothing like the movie in our class. As soon as he latched on, he went right to sleep and I know he didn't get anything because he barely sucked."*

LC: *"So are you saying that the first feeding didn't go well because he appeared to be sleeping instead of actively feeding?"*

Active listening will also help the LC remove herself from her own perception of emotions and allow the mother to articulate how she feels about a given situation. This will enable the LC to better serve the mother's needs and open the door for more difficult topics, if needed.

Example: The mother may say, *"The first feeding is supposed to be the most important one, but all the baby did was fall asleep without sucking."* The LC can focus on the words "supposed to," as well as the mother's tone of voice in her response by stating, *"It sounds like you feel that your baby isn't doing well."*

Supportive Communication

Supportive communication is particularly helpful when the mother appears frustrated or needs to be understood. This can come in the form of reassurance, such as "I am glad you decided to offer supplement since the baby had not eaten in so many hours. The first rule is always to feed the baby." Reassurance can strengthen the professional bond between the mother and the LC, making her feel that she isn't being judged. For this technique to be effective, reassurance must be valid; pat phrases are easily identified and can lead to lost trust.

Another form of supportive communication is empathy. Empathy is recognition and response to a patient's feelings without criticism

(Swartz, 1998). True empathy allows the mother to feel less isolated, understand that her problem is real and recognized, and that she is not alone. Empathy can be given in a simple statement, such as "It sounds like you are frustrated after seeing the first feeding look so easy in the movie, when your experience turned out so differently." It is up to the LC to probe further, using empathy as a communication tool, in order to accurately identify what the mother is trying to express emotionally. For example, she may be verbalizing about her lack of help at a hospital, but internalizing guilt because her baby got formula from a bottle during her stay. If the LC focuses solely on possible anger and frustration, or worse still, shares that this is something that she herself gets aggravated over, she will miss that the mother is really feeling guilty or ashamed. This is generally not the time for the LC to share her own breastfeeding challenges, something that can be tempting to do with this technique. The focus must remain on the mother and baby.

Confrontation

Although confrontation has a negative connotation, in the context of communication techniques, it describes a method for clarifying inconsistencies with data. This communication style is generally given as a direct question, frequently pointing out the inconsistency. The mother is often unaware of the inconsistency. The direct question acts as a prompt, generally when she is recounting an event.

Example: "When you filled out your history form, you wrote that the baby eats every three hours and has one five hour sleep period in 24 hours. You also wrote that he gets a total of eight feedings in 24 hours. These numbers only add up to six or seven feedings in 24 hours. Do you have these feedings written down somewhere?"

When confrontation is used, delivery must be calm, non-judgmental, and simply questioning. It is very easy to put a mother on the defensive with this technique, leading to a decrease or even halt in the flow of information. Confrontation should be used in a very limited capacity and not necessarily with all mothers.

Branching Questions

The term "branching questions" may not be commonly recognized, but it is an often used interviewing technique. When used, the LC typically focuses on a newly identified problem for further assessment and to work toward the plan.

Example: Pain is the most common reason for breastfeeding problems and early weaning. However, pain assessment can be complex due to many variables, most of which area based on the mother's response. Figure Two is an example of branching questions for brief pain assessment during the history interview only. Based on the mother's verbal and non verbal responses, further questioning and a full feeding assessment is still necessary.

Mother's Non-verbal Response	Interview Question: Pain	Mother's Verbal Response
Calm, introspective	When do you typically feel pain?	During a feeding, after a feeding, etc.
May make a face, shoulders curve inward	What does your pain feel like?	Often descriptive terms such as burning, stabbing, shooting, pinching, and so on.
Calm, reflective; may still have protective posturing	What do you do to avoid or relieve your pain?	Breaking the latch, hydrogel dressings, milk expression, lanolin, etc. Typically a stated intervention.
May appear confused, discouraged, or angry	Does this work?	Response will probably be fairly negative since she is seeking additional help.
May appear tired and discouraged	How long has this pain been occurring?	Usually a stated time interval
May have reflexive body movement	Do you have any other symptoms along with pain?	Can have nausea as a pain response. May also describe skin changes, tissue changes, or other health systems that are impacted.
May become teary, particularly if problem is leading to some depression. Conversely, if mother is stoic, affect may appear flat.	Are you having any difficulties with postpartum adjustment or self care as a result of your pain?	Pace of verbal flow may speed up or slow down, depending on mother's emotional state. The stoic mother may answer with less detail.

Figure 2: Branching Questions

Nonverbal Cue Observation

It is important to observe body language and nonverbal cues. However, body language is not a stand-alone form of communication. Arm crossing or leaning back is thought to be typical avoidance movements or negative communication, but they may also indicate that the individual is cold, or they may be a character trait.

Frequent movement or position change can communicate some degree of discomfort. The LC response to this would be to ask directly "are you uncomfortable with this question or is something else bothering you?" The mother may be too polite or shy to bring up whatever issue is uppermost in her mind at that time, so it is the role of the LC to draw her out rather than overlooking it.

Nonverbal observation is especially helpful during a feeding assessment. The mother may not report pain because she is waiting for it to pass, assumes it is normal, or is expecting the LC to be aware of it already. "Toe-curling pain" is a descriptive, but very applicable phrase, since this is a common non-verbal cue that mothers demonstrate. In addition, back stiffening, hunching, or involuntary pulling away are also good indicators of pain.

Secondary Sources of Communication

In many instances, when recounting events such as labor or feedings right after delivery, it is helpful to have the mother's partner or other support persons present for their input as well, but only with her consent. Family and support persons are a great resource. They often observe the mother's reactions to feeding difficulties without the mother realizing it. They may also have their own anxieties regarding the breastfeeding process, which, if left unaddressed, can undermine the implementation of a plan or breastfeeding all together. Having a support person present for a consultation can also help ensure that information and education given to the mother is correctly received. A support person who is engaged in the breastfeeding process will act as a means of ongoing positive reinforcement, something that the LC is unable to do at the same level.

Members of the healthcare team are an excellent source of data for history collection. This is everyone from physicians to a nurse tech. In the inpatient setting, the greatest individual source of information is the staff nurse who is typically with the mother and/or baby for at least twelve hours. In addition to documentation in the medical record, staff nurses communicate by report, given verbally at shift changes. The report may be given in a group setting or nurse to nurse, based on patient assignments and practice settings; this varies by organization. Shift report generally includes:

- Name and location/room number
- Allergies
- Vital signs
- Current medications
- Current health status
- Current or recent health complications while hospitalized
- Problems or concerns
- Expected date of discharge
- Shift details, identified needs

ILCs should attempt to be present for the report or at least obtain a basic shift report from the primary care nurse and should note additional or subjective details on the history form. Because ILCs have many patients within one shift, an informal tool to use for the report is a tickler or worksheet. The worksheet is not part of the medical record, but rather a place for the ILC to make brief notes, as well as keep pertinent details straight regarding a variety of patients. Because it contains private health information, the sheet should be destroyed at the end of the shift or after use.

If a referral is made to the PPLC from a doctor's office, clinic, or hospital, it is helpful to obtain a brief verbal report from the referral source. Many times, the referral comes from the physician or midwife, but it is called in by a triage or office nurse who may not have been present during the actual appointment. The PPLC can ask the nurse to read the progress notes by phone or to transmit if a confidential fax is available.

> *Teaching Tip: When the significant other, family member, or support person is present, it is important to ask them specifically if they have any questions or concerns. They may bring up issues the mother forgot to ask about or be uncomfortable mentioning.*

Chapter Three

MATERNAL HISTORY

Structure

To take an accurate patient history, several items must be included. Initially, the history begins with the mother, since before delivery, she and the baby are considered one entity. However, after delivery, the history will begin to overlap, and then expand out, so that the baby has his own history. The LC should consolidate all of this information onto one documentation tool, but there should be separate areas on the tool for mother and baby.

For the ILC, most, if not all, of the mother's medical history, along with the birth history, will already be present in the medical record or chart. It will probably be spread out in different sections: pregnancy details on faxed forms from the obstetrical caregiver, demographics on a face sheet, the birth process on a labor record or even recorded solely on monitor strips. The baby's information will probably be in a separate record, likely in a different location. It is the responsibility of the ILC to complete a full history review before seeing the patient.

For the outpatient or PPLC, the history may be completed in advance by telephone or by the mother upon receiving the form from email or fax. It should be reviewed by the LC with the mother before proceeding.

Biography

The biography refers to the baseline information and is generically called the demographics. Most of the demographics are usually on the first page of the electronic or physical medical record. They are often the first section of an outpatient style history form. Demographics start with the mother's basic contact information:

- Home address
- Phone number
- The mother's date of birth
- Marital status
- Husband or partner's name
- Husband or partner's contact information if different

Age is an important factor, not only for communication style and techniques, but also for values, beliefs, and perceptions of the mother. The Generation X mother will have different goals and viewpoints from the Generation Y or teen mother. Each will require individualization; therefore, it is probably beneficial to list the mother's age in addition to date of birth in order to ensure better support.

Although race is often included on a face sheet of a hospital record, the LC should probably avoid using this as part of her demographic information. The race categories set up by the U.S. Census Bureau can often be misleading, and accuracy for the individual based on this listing is dependent on the knowledge and training of the interviewer. For example, Haitians are categorized as "black" because "West Indian" is often not on the form. Even when self-completed, errors can occur, such as a Brazilian who checks "white" because Hispanic (Spain/Spanish) is inaccurate. Families with blended cultures present a whole new difficulty with categorization (Lipson et al., 2002). The LC is better off asking open-ended questions regarding belief systems, family and community traditions, and cultural practices.

The lactation consultant who will have continued interaction with a patient (such as postpartum calls, warm line assistance, follow-up appointments, or even online support) will need to obtain additional information. This will include a patient's cell phone number and personal email address. In the case of a teen mother living with a parent, the name of a close relative with telephone contact may also be helpful, but be sure to obtain permission from the mother to contact the relative.

Because of IBLCE Scope of Practice standards (IBCLE, 2008) to "work collaboratively and interdependently with other members of the healthcare team," the LC will need the name of the mother's primary caregiver. Getting the primary caregiver's contact phone number is very time saving, particularly for the outpatient or private practice LC. If the mother attends a large group practice, the name of the delivering physician or midwife should be listed and reports sent to their attention when necessary.

Demographic details for the LC will also include the baby's identifying information. This includes the baby's full name (including last), date of birth, and primary caregiver, with phone number. In some instances the baby may be attended by multiple caregivers, particularly in the military setting. If this is the case, list the referring caregiver or head of the practice. Location of the baby after delivery is important for all LCs to know. If the baby went to a

NICU or was transferred to another facility for a higher level of care, this will definitely impact the breastfeeding experience, regardless of resolution. The same applies to the mother who experiences complications during or after labor and may require a high level of care as a result.

In some practice environments, it is important to note primary spoken and written language. If English is a second language, it is critical to assess fluency, as well as identify if the patient can read English. If the patient is not fluent and brings an interpreter, English fluency of the interpreter must also be assessed, unless the interpreter is hired by an agency for medical purposes.

Additionally, if insurance is filed for the consultation, this information is collected with the demographics. Generally, this includes the insurers name, group number, and policy number. If the primary insured is someone other than the mother, such as her husband, it is also important to collect his date of birth and social security number. For billing and filing purposes, it is a good idea to make a photocopy of the insurance card, as the card contains contact information for the insurance company.

A helpful, but not always directly necessary detail is the mother's employment status, even if she is leaving the workforce to stay home, or if she is in school. Each of these situations can present specific challenges not only to breastfeeding, but also to transition to parenthood in general. The ILC will rarely address transition to workplace needs while making daily rounds, but a note on the medical record will aid future support calls or outpatient consultations.

> *Teaching Tip:* Demographic information can give the LC possible clues about the mother's culture or environment of support, but only if she has a good familiarity with the resources and characteristics of her practice community. For example, a mother who has a home address located on the site of a military base may be able to access a Soldier and Family Readiness program. These programs often provide classes, support groups, and other resources for new parents.

Reason for Consult

The purpose behind the consultation should be listed fairly early on the history form. In the inpatient setting, it may be routine for all breastfeeding patients to be assessed, but this should still be noted. However, in all settings, if the mother is seen for a problem, this should be detailed in the mother's words, rather than just a one line statement. Physicians refer to this as the "chief complaint." Detailed information includes how long the mother has been experiencing the problem and any impact on herself, her baby, or the family. The LC should identify when the problem started and whether the problem has gotten worse.

Also noted should be the referring source, as well as any other individuals who are assisting the mother specifically with breastfeeding. This doesn't include family members who are present in the home to help with mother and baby care, unless they are providing breastfeeding advice and assessment.

By stating the purpose for the consult early on the history form, the LC is better able to identify potential concerns that may relate to the problem as she reviews the history. Even if the identified problem is different from the initial reason for the consult, this aids in a more complete assessment.

Health

A physician, midwife, or nurse's health history contains a review of each body system, and all three approaches are very similar. However, this style is generally more detailed than the LC needs. To obtain an overview of the mother's general health as it relates to breastfeeding, it is easier to create a simple checklist of common medical conditions or issues that may impact lactation, looking for variations from the norm. Because so many of these issues can also impact pregnancy, the inpatient LC can often find them listed on the prenatal records sent from the doctor's office to be placed in the medical record.

If the mother's history is obtained by interview or if the LC needs additional details, it is advisable to ask all family members to step out of the room, unless the mother requests otherwise. Many elements of the health history can be sensitive to the mother, and there may be some details she hasn't shared, even with a husband or partner. By assuming that all information is private, the mother is not put in the position of asking her family to leave, and she is more likely to be forthcoming when alone. Again, it is critical for the LC to appear matter of fact and non-judgmental during a health history interview.

Health issues that can potentially impact breastfeeding can be easily listed in a check box format, with additional space for details when answered in the affirmative. If the form is sent to the patient electronically, it should be stressed on a cover sheet, email, or the form itself that all health information will be kept confidential and not discussed when family members are present, unless the mother desires otherwise.

Common health issues can include, but are not limited to:

• Smoking
- How many cigarettes are smoked per day or week?
- How long has she been a smoker?
- Did she smoke during pregnancy?
- Has she ever tried to quit either on her own or through a formal program?

• Alcohol use
- Is she a social or occasional drinker verses a regular drinker?
- If regular, state volume per day, week, or month
- Has alcohol use ever been a problem or concern to her?
- Was there any use during pregnancy?

• Depression
- Has she ever been diagnosed with clinical depression?
- Is she currently being treated; if so, how?
- Does she have a current mental health caregiver?
- List name and contact information
- If not currently treated, how long since her last treatment?
- Was depression ongoing or event specific?

• Panic or Anxiety Disorder
- Has she ever been clinically diagnosed?
- Is she currently being treated; if so, how?
- Does she have a current mental health caregiver?
- List name and contact information
- If not currently treated, how long since last treatment?
- Was the panic disorder ongoing or event specific?

• Infertility
- Was a reason identified?
- Did she have a full fertility workup including any exploratory surgery?
- Any variations found in hormone levels?
- How did this pregnancy occur?

• Breast Surgery
- Type of surgery
- When was it performed?

- Were there any complications?
- Was there any discussion with the surgeon regarding future breastfeeding options?
• Pregnancy Loss, Abortion (on the prenatal record as SAB, EAB)
   - How many pregnancies has she had?
   - How far along were her losses?
   - How many medical or elective abortions?
• Diabetes
   - Identify her age at diagnosis
   - Type of diabetes and current treatment
   - How well was her diabetes controlled during pregnancy?
   (This will not include gestational diabetes which is addressed later.)
• Thyroid disorders
   - Identify type and when diagnosed
   - Current or past treatments
   - Any medical complications relating to diagnosis?
• Pituitary disorder
   - Identify type and when diagnosed
   - Current or past treatments
   - Any medical complications relating to diagnosis?
• Polycystic Ovarian Syndrome (PCOS)
   - Identify any issues related to syndrome
   - Any medical complications related to syndrome?
• Food Allergies
   -Differentiate between sensitivity and actual allergies
      -Type of reaction, when it started, family history
• Medication Allergies
   - Medication type
   - Reaction response
   - When allergy was first identified
   (Often patient will mistake a common reaction, such as nausea, for an allergy.)
• Physical, Emotional or Sexual Abuse
   - Age when abuse started; type?
   - If the abuse was sexual, has the mother experienced any trigger responses to labor, birth, or breastfeeding?
      - Could current breastfeeding problem be related to past abuse?

Once the primary health issues have been identified and addressed, the mother should be asked if there are any other ongoing medical issues. Often, this is where problems such as high blood pressure or arthritis are discussed. Although many ongoing medical conditions will not relate specifically to a breastfeeding problem requiring consultation, the patient will still need support regarding medication safety and tips for dealing with related challenges.

Example: A mother with rheumatoid arthritis who experiences a flair-up may already be aware of medication safety, but may need support with alternate positioning and fatigue. Information on this can be provided at the end of a consultation or in a follow up call or email.

The LC will want to know about any other major surgeries (aside from breast), according to type and when performed. Minor or childhood surgeries, such as wisdom teeth or tonsils, are not clinically relevant and do not need detailing.

Diet

The mother's diet is important to assess in the interview. Most mothers feel a little defensive about having a nutritionally erratic diet during the postpartum period, so it is important to reassure her while offering suggestions for improving the diet if needed. Typically, simple encouragement regarding basic nutrition is all that is necessary.

A mother who is vegetarian, vegan, or practices alternative diet therapies should be further evaluated. Vegetarians may eat eggs, fish or both; vegans eat only plant foods. Length of the current dietary preferences and food requirements during lactation should be reviewed. Concerns about inadequacies are usually vitamin or mineral focused, such as B^{12} or iron. This issue can be addressed by suggesting the mother add vitamin supplements, fortified soy milk, fortified yeast, whole grains, and legumes to her diet. If a need is identified, the LC can refer the mother to a dietician for further counseling and education.

If the mother is eating or avoiding special or cultural foods to assist with birth recovery or milk production, it is helpful to note this as well, not only to better support the mother, but also to increase the LC's knowledge base. In many cultures both in and outside of the U.S., mothers have used foods for health purposes for generations. Some have become mainstream, such as oatmeal for increasing milk production or yogurt with live acidophilus cultures to prevent yeast. Because of increasing global awareness, the LC should be aware of cross cultural foods that are becoming mainstream. One that is currently eliciting much interest for milk production is Shatavari. The root is commonly found in India and is used to brew a tea for lactating mothers. Women from many places in South America will brew a drink primarily from a sugar called Panela, also to increase their supply.

> *Teaching Tip: Some faiths, such as Muslim, practice fasting during certain events or time frames. Often the pregnant or lactating mother is exempt from fasting. But if she is not, she can be educated on high energy foods to prepare for the fast or to eat when the fast is over. She can also be encouraged to reduce her physical activity during the fast to reduce her caloric demand.*

Drugs and Herbs

Any current medications that the mother is taking, whether regularly or as needed (prn), should be noted. Compatibility to breastfeeding should be verified by the LC using lactation specific resources, such as LactMed or *Medications and Mother's Milk* (Hale, 2008), particularly with medications she doesn't recognize or is uncertain about. It should not be assumed that medication safety has been confirmed by the primary caregiver or pharmacist.

The LC should ask about vitamin supplements, herbal supplements, medicinal herbs, and any natural remedies. Often mothers will try herbal remedies, thinking they are innocuous, when they can actually have as great an effect as medication - potentially greater since herbal manufacturing is a less regulated industry (Humphries, 2003). Mothers can also mistake the potential potency of an herb when used to excess.

Example: Some mothers drink multiple cups of peppermint tea throughout the day for digestion and relaxation. However, peppermint oil can actually reduce milk production. The mother may need education regarding this, as well as help identifying an alternate remedy.

This topic provides an opening for the discussion of recreational drug use. Although the majority of breastfeeding women probably do not use illegal or recreational drugs, there are some who will. The most dangerous of these drugs are probably heroin, cocaine, and crack, which readily cross the milk cell barrier for the baby to ingest. There are documented cases of babies who have had serious reactions to exposure to these drugs; therefore, the mother who continues or resumes use of these drugs should not breastfeed. In addition, the mother who uses illegal or recreational drugs is probably putting her infant at a safety risk, at the very least. Implications for mandatory reporting in her state should be investigated by the LC.

Methadone used by recovering heroin addicts is considered compatible with breastfeeding.

Complementary Therapies

If the mother receives current complementary therapies or has accessed these in the past, it may be helpful to use these as a resource for any current problems. Complementary therapy information can be easily listed in a check box format, with space given to identify anything unfamiliar to the LC. Examples include:

- Chiropractic
- Acupuncture
- Acupressure
- Cranio sacral therapy (CST)
- Massage therapy
- Rolfing
- Herbals

It may be helpful to obtain contact information for the complimentary therapist or caregiver, not only for mother-baby support, but also for the LC to build her own resource list and knowledge base in less familiar areas.

Additional Children

If the patient has other children, their names, sex, ages, and any breastfeeding history should be noted. Blended families present challenges that can impact breastfeeding, so non-biological children present in the home should also be listed. Discussing the mother's breastfeeding experience with a previous child or children can give the LC information that may help with the current problem, particularly if the mother had an unsuccessful breastfeeding experience.

The LC should not assume that the mother's perception of her previous problem is a fully accurate representation of the feeding issue. Many mothers are given misinformation from individuals who do not have evidence-based knowledge of breastfeeding or were not part of the mother's breastfeeding care, and as a result may be unaware of the actual cause. Discussion of the previous breastfeeding experience may bring up some unresolved grief. This was most likely a stressful and unhappy time, and she is very likely to have continued dissatisfaction with the outcome. Many mothers blame themselves for an unsuccessful breastfeeding experience and may secretly believe that there is something wrong with their body or mothering behavior. Time should be allowed for them to tell their story.

Example: Often a mother will come to the LC before having her second baby because she was told that she couldn't make milk with her first child. Evidence shows that she probably didn't have good support and education, which can lead to a low supply, possibly related to early supplementation and/ or inadequate stimulation. The mother must first be reassured on this point before she can move forward.

Pregnancy History

The mother's pregnancy experience can provide many clues regarding breastfeeding issues. The LC should first identify if the mother experienced normal pregnancy changes in her breasts. Often, simply asking the mother if she had changes is not enough. The LC should specifically ask about size increase, darkening of the nipple, and leaking during pregnancy. Other changes that may not be as quickly recognized are prominence of veins, the skin seems thinner, Montgomery glands enlarge, and breasts appear tender or more sensitive. If the mother seems anxious about little or no changes, reassurance about individuality should be offered.

Pregnancy complications should be explored. If the complications were severe, breastfeeding may be impacted. Not only may the infant be immature due to an early or induced delivery, but the mother may also have fewer emotional or physical resources. If she was on bed rest for several weeks or longer, she may have increased fatigue due to a loss of stamina and even some muscle atrophy. If she had preeclampsia or other maternal complications, feedings may have been initially delayed, or she may have fatigue and inability to focus due to medication therapy.

Prenatal Education

Prenatal education is important; a mother who is well educated has a greater chance at breastfeeding success. Good versus poor prenatal education is getting more difficult to measure with increased dependency on the Internet and the rapid changes within the economy and the healthcare system. Current research shows that fewer women are taking prenatal education classes and are opting to use the Internet and books instead. The perception is that traditional prenatal classes are dated, "something their mothers did," and are unnecessary for this generation (Declercq et al., 2007).

If the mother attended classes, identify which classes she took and who attended them with her. Not all classes are the same in content and quality. Many birth classes that used to teach breastfeeding as part of the curriculum no longer offer this. In addition, the majority of women who attend prenatal classes do so at the facility where they plan to give birth. As a result of critical nursing shortages, classes are often taught by poorly trained ancillary staff, where course curriculum has remained unchanged over the years with the single exception of decreasing classroom hours.

If the mother has been reading or visiting websites, ask for specifics. The LC should be familiar with all prenatal classes in her area, with a general knowledge of the curriculum and focus. She should also have a working knowledge of the most commonly accessed websites for prenatal education by parents.

The mother should also be asked about parenting classes, programs, or books. Unlike traditional prenatal classes, parenting classes are on the rise and are attended either before or after the baby is born. They are often held in non-traditional settings, such as a church or synagogue, recreation center, or wellness facility. Some popular parenting curriculums that recommend structured feedings or scheduling can impact lactation significantly.

Birth Information

The labor information can be obtained from the medical record, but the specific details are far better obtained by the patient interview. If the father or birth partner is present for this, it is a help for the mother who may not be able to recount specifics, particularly if she received IV pain medications.

It is important to learn about the birth setting. The ILC will have an understanding of birth practices within her workplace, but the outpatient or PPLC should be familiar with common practices at all of the local birth environments. In addition, if home birth is available in the area, the LC should make a point of meeting with area midwives whenever possible to become familiar with this birth practice, as well.

Basic information should include gestational age by week at the time of delivery. In addition, the labor process itself is very important. This includes how labor began, any medications associated with labor, such as Cytotec, prostaglandins, or Pitocin, side effects of any of these medications, and how long labor lasted. If labor was induced, it is important to note if the mother was already experiencing any signs of labor beforehand.

If the mother received pain medication during labor, the LC should note the type of medication, how it was administered, and how much was taken. If the mother had an epidural, the LC should note how long the medication was infused and if there were any problems related to the epidural or other pain medications. This will include the need to reposition, increase the dosage, or replace the epidural for incomplete or ineffective coverage.

Birth information should include the time of delivery. The LC can ask how long the mother pushed. If the vaginal birth was assisted by forceps or vacuum, this should be noted as well, and the infant assessed for trauma. If the mother delivered by cesarean section, it should be differentiated by emergent or planned, and the documented or patient stated rationale for the cesarean section. In addition, the LC should note the type of anesthesia used for the cesarean section.

The mother should be asked about any difficulties or complications regarding the labor process or any problems afterward in the recovery phase and initial postpartum period. This is specific to her only; infant complications will be addressed later. The mother should be asked about postpartum bleeding: if it seemed too heavy or she passed a lot of clots. The inpatient LC will be able to identify volume lost and associated medications from the medical record, the outpatient or PPLC will need to rely on the mother as the historian. The LC should ask if the patient received blood or blood products, Methergine, and if the mother knows her hemoglobin levels.

Finally, the mother should be questioned about postpartum pain and bleeding. She has already listed her medications, but if the consult occurs within the first two weeks, the amount and frequency of medications may be applicable to breastfeeding issues, although not necessarily through into-milk transmission.

Depression

During the course of the history, particularly during the interview, the LC may recognize some potential indicators of depression. This most commonly occurs in the Outpatient or PPLC setting. Many times, when a mother has requested breastfeeding support, the LC is the first professional to recognize symptoms of Postpartum Depression. Risk factors include:

- History of clinical depression
- Pregnancy complications or unplanned outcomes
- Lack of social support

Rates of postpartum depression vary widely, but on average, seem to be about 15-20%. Unless the LC is also a physician, she cannot diagnose this medical condition. However, if she identifies a mother with this possibility, she can further assess by administering the Edinburgh Postnatal Depression Scale (EPDS) (Cox et al., 1987), a risk assessment tool developed to help identify mothers who are experiencing these difficulties (Attachment E). Copies of the EPDS should be sent to the primary caregiver, regardless of results in order to maintain continuity. If the mother indicates that she has considered harming herself, her primary caregiver should be contacted immediately.

Attachment E

The EPDS Risk Assessment Tool to Support the History Assessment

EDINBURGH POSTNATAL DEPRESSION SCALE (EPDS)

The EPDS was developed for screening postpartum women in outpatient, home visiting settings, or at the six to eight week postpartum examination. It has been utilized among numerous populations, including U.S. women and Spanish speaking women in other countries.

The EPDS consists of ten questions. The test can usually be completed in less than five minutes. Responses are scored 0, 1, 2, or 3 according to increased severity of the symptom. Items marked with an asterisk (*) are reverse scored (i.e., 3, 2, 1, and 0). The total score is determined by adding together the scores for each of the ten items.

Validation studies have utilized various threshold scores in determining which women were positive and in need of referral. Cut-off scores ranged from 9 to 13 points. Therefore, to err on safety's side, a woman scoring 9 or more points or indicating any suicidal ideation – that is she scores 1 or higher on question #10 – should be referred immediately for follow-up.

Even if a woman scores less than 9, if the clinician feels the client is suffering from depression, an appropriate referral should be made. The EPDS is only a screening tool. It does not diagnose depression – that is done by appropriately licensed health care personnel. Users may reproduce the scale without permission, providing the copyright is respected by quoting the names of the authors, title, and source of the paper in all reproduced copies.

Instructions for Users:
1. The mother is asked to underline one of four possible responses that comes the closest to how she has been feeling the previous seven days.
2. All ten items must be completed.
3. Care should be taken to avoid the possibility of the mother discussing her answers with others.
4. The mother should complete the scale herself, unless she has limited English or difficulty reading.

EPDS/Postpartum Risk Assessment

Name:_____

Date:_____ **Address:** _____

Baby's Name: _____ **Baby's Age:** _____

As you have recently had a baby, we would like to know how you are feeling. Please UNDERLINE the answer which comes closest to how you have felt IN THE PAST 7 DAYS, not just how you feel today. Here is an example, already completed.

> *I have felt happy:*
> ❑ *Yes, all the time*
> ❑ <u>*Yes, most of the time*</u>
> ❑ *No, not very often*
> ❑ *No, not at all*

This would mean: "I have felt happy most of the time" during the past week. Please complete the other questions in the same way.

In the past 7 days:

1. I have been able to laugh and see the funny side of things.
   - ❑ As much as I always could
   - ❑ Not quite so much now
   - ❑ Not at all

2. I have looked forward with enjoyment to things.
   - ❑ As much as I ever did
   - ❑ Rather less than I used to
   - ❑ Definitely less than I used to
   - ❑ Hardly at all

*3. I have blamed myself unnecessarily when things went wrong.
   - ❑ Yes, most of the time
   - ❑ Yes, some of the time
   - ❑ Not very often
   - ❑ No, never

4. I have been anxious or worried for no good reason.

      ◻ No, not at all

      ◻ Hardly ever

      ◻ Yes, sometimes

      ◻ Yes, very often

*5. I have felt scared or panicky for no very good reason.

      ◻ Yes, quite a lot

      ◻ Yes, sometimes

      ◻ No, not much

      ◻ No, not at all

*6. Things have been getting on top of me.

      ◻ Yes, most of the time I haven't been able to cope at all

      ◻ Yes, sometimes I haven't been coping as well as usual

      ◻ No, most of the time I have coped quite well

      ◻ No, have been coping as well as ever

*7. I have been so unhappy that I have had difficulty sleeping.

      ◻ Yes, most of the time

      ◻ Yes, sometimes

      ◻ Not very often

      ◻ No, not at all

*8. I have felt sad or miserable.

      ◻ Yes, most of the time

      ◻ Yes, quite often

      ◻ Not very often

      ◻ No, not at all

*9 I have been so unhappy that I have been crying.

      ◻ Yes, most of the time

      ◻ Yes, quite often

      ◻ Only occasionally

      ◻ No, never

*10. The thought of harming myself has occurred to me.

      ◻ Yes, quite often

      ◻ Sometimes

      ◻ Hardly ever

      ◻ Never

Cox JL, Holden JM, Sagovsky R. Detection of postnatal depression. Development of the 10-item Edinburgh Postnatal Depression Scale. *Br J Psychiatry*. 1987. 150:782-86.

Chapter Four

NEWBORN AND FEEDING HISTORY

Newborn/Infant History

The natural flow from maternal health, pregnancy, and birth is to focus on the newborn. Again, most of the documentation and attention is given to variations from the norm or factors that can impact breastfeeding.

Postpartum Transition

If the baby experienced any difficulties with transition or other problems after delivery, these should be explored further. For the ILC, this can be a method for identifying at risk newborns needing early follow up. For the outpatient or PPLC, this can provide direction for identifying problems. If the newborn is in a traditional hospital environment and the baby was held in the nursery for longer than one to two hours, the ILC should talk to the Nursery staff about transition issues - was the baby being observed for some reason? Sometimes a nurse will just have a "gut feeling" that the baby doesn't seem to be transitioning well, although there may be only subtle indicators. Babies who are directly admitted to the NICU or Special Care Nursery should have documentation identifying rationale for admission and any complications.

At the very least, the APGAR score should be noted to determine how well the baby transitioned through labor. Although it is not to be used as any sort of predictor for well-being, it can serve as an additional information piece in the history process. The scoring is completed at one and five minutes postpartum, with additional assessment for a total score of less than seven.

	Sign	0 Points	1 Point	2 Points
A	Activity (Muscle Tone)	Absent	Arms and legs flexed	Active movement
P	Pulse	Absent	Below 100 bpm	Above 100 bpm
G	Grimace (reflex irritability)	No response	Grimace	Sneeze, coughs, pulls away
A	Appearance (skin color)	Blue-gray, pale all over	Normal, except for extremities	Normal over entire body
R	Respiration	Absent	Slow, irregular	Good, crying

Figure 3. An example of a basic APGAR Scoring System; an expanded version is currently used for Neonatal Resuscitation Procedure (AAP, 2006).

Maturity Scoring

The baby's estimated gestational age is determined by the mother's menses and pregnancy ultrasound. Often, the first ultrasound is done at eight weeks in order to get the most accurate determination of age possible. However, even though ultrasound machines and technicians have improved greatly over the years, there is still a variance allowance of about ten to eleven days, which can mean the difference between preterm, near term, and full term.

There are several scoring tools that can be administered by healthcare professionals within the first few hours after delivery in order to better identify actual gestational age. The best known are the Dubowitz Method and the New Ballard Score. These two assessment tools are maturity ratings primarily centered on neuromuscular development and reflexes. The ratings are assigned by staff nurses or pediatricians within the first few hours after delivery. The ratings are extremely helpful for determining gestational age, unless the baby is very ill or extremely premature. They are two separate assessments; although sometimes, they are referred to interchangeably or together. When the two numbers for gestational age by exam and age by date are varied, this may help identify some of the potential reasons for feeding and suck issues.

Not all healthcare facilities routinely perform these assessments. The LC should be aware of organizational practices in her work environment and community if she has this question as part of her history form. The mother may not be familiar with this assessment, even if it was performed, so the ILC may need to define it for her, as well as assist with locating results on a discharge form. The outpatient or PPLC can contact the pediatric office, as these results should be on information sent after delivery from the hospital or birth center for the baby's medical record.

The First Feedings

The first feeding should be well documented as far as time and mother's impression. If the mother thinks the feedings aren't going well, it often doesn't matter how well the observer reports that they went (Dunn et al., 2006).

If the baby was supplemented in the early days after delivery, the LC should identify:

- Rationale-indicators for supplement with supportive data
- Type-expressed colostrum, formula, glucose water
- Method-syringe, bottle, cup, finger feeding, SNS
- Infant response-if noted in the record, how well the baby tolerated the feeding

In addition, if any feeding tool was introduced, this should also be noted, with rationale if possible. If supplement is offered more than once, the mother should have started pumping, typically initiated by the nursing staff. The ILC should review the nurse's notes to ensure that the mother received instructions on pump setup, frequency, and duration, as well as care and cleaning of all parts. If it appears that the mother will need to continue pumping, she should have been given a list of rental stations in the area. Generally, this is a part of the patient education resources available in nurse's stations or some other central, accessible location. Most hospitals require a variety of vendors to be listed whenever possible to meet corporate compliance standards.

Post Discharge

For the hospital-born infant without complications, the LC should note if the mother roomed in, requested demand feedings, or sent the baby to the nursery at night or for naps. The LC will need to clarify this for the entire hospital stay. If the baby was born at a birth center and discharge home was delayed or the baby and mother were transferred to a hospital, the LC should identify the rationale.

At this point, the history is complete for the ILC. The OLC and PPLC should continue with a review of feedings and maternal and infant health up to the point of the consultation. This will include:

- Current age by day or week
- Date and rationale for first pediatric caregiver visit

- If followed for jaundice,
  - include bilirubin levels
  - treatments administered with duration
- If followed for excessive weight loss
  - include all weights with dates
  - determine percentage of loss from birth
  - document all supplements by type, method, and duration
- Stooling in past 24 hours
  - number, amount, and color
- Wet Diapers
  - number, color of urine
- Number of breastfeedings in the past 24 hours
  - Does the baby show hunger cues "before it's time to feed"?
- Longest sleep period in the past 24 hours
  - Does the baby have to be awakened for feedings?
  - Where does the baby typically sleep?

The OLC or PPLC should also determine if the baby had a full feeding assessment by an ILC or knowledgeable breastfeeding support person. Often, a mother may have had a visit by the "breastfeeding person," but only part of a feeding may have been observed, or possibly no feeding at all.

> *Teaching Tip: A discussion of gestational age, along with age by exam if available, provides an opportunity to educate the patient about the differences between preterm, near term, and full term. This can help the mother set realistic goals based on her infant's actual, rather than preconceived, capabilities.*

Breastfeeding History

Output should be identified, particularly stooling. Many parents are under the impression that wet diapers are a single, accurate evaluation of intake. A review of stooling patterns provides an opportunity for patient education (Nommsen-Rivers et al., 2008). Bowel movements for the previous 24 hours should be tracked according to frequency, an estimation of amount, and color. Parents can be educated on the differences between meconium, bilirubin excretion, and normal breastmilk stools. If the infant isn't stooling well, wet diapers should also be assessed for frequency, urine color, and an estimation of volume.

The mother should be asked about feeding frequency and duration. Many mothers will automatically answer "every two to three hours." If they have been tracking feedings, the LC can ask to see their notes or form. The LC may need to spend some time discussing and identifying what constitutes an actual feeding. She may also need to define feeding duration as the time the baby spends nutritively suckling at the breast, rather than including the time for burping, diaper changes, and waking the baby. If the baby has one or more long sleep periods within a 24 hour time frame, this can also impact the number of feedings without the mother accounting for it.

Supplemental Feedings/Pumping
If the mother is supplementing feedings, the LC must document the type, volume, and how it is given. If this is different from the initial plan made either in the hospital or at a previous visit, this should be noted. The mother can be asked how she feels the baby is tolerating the supplemental feedings.

If the mother is pumping, noted will be the pump brand and type, settings she is using, frequency, and duration. An average volume of expressed milk should also be documented. If she has a personal use pump, the LC should determine if it was purchased new by this mother, as opposed to previously owned. Shared single user pumps are becoming more widespread and present potential problems. In addition to infection risk, the efficiency of the pump diminishes over time, potentially impacting the mother's supply. Effective pumping should be further addressed during the assessment phase.

History Conclusion
At this point, it is helpful to ask open-ended questions about anything that is unclear or if there are additional details the mother thinks you should know. Throughout the verbal history, but especially during the discussion of feedings, the mother and her support person's knowledge base regarding breastfeeding should be analyzed.

A discussion of the patient's current breastfeeding goals, short term as well as long term, will allow the LC to better meet the mother's needs. This final discussion will then allow the assessment process to begin.

Chapter Five

PHYSICAL ASSESSMENT

Physical assessment consists of three things: the mother, the baby, and the feeding. Documentation of the mother and baby should continue to be variations from the norm; however, documentation of the feeding should be observations and impressions. The history form is a helpful tool to use as a starting point for assessment. Additionally, it is a guide for further evaluation of variations.

Tools that can help with assessment:
- Penlight
  - For visualizing the inside of the baby's mouth, tongue movement, and palate.
- Vinyl gloves
  - Latex will sensitize and put the baby at risk for allergy
  - PPLCs who do home visits may not be aware of a latex allergy in advance
- Gauze
  - For wiping a coated tongue
  - May help with mobility assessment
- Measuring tape
  - For detailing a wound or inflammation
- Scale
  - Two gram accuracy; if portable, LC should calibrate weight and check accuracy regularly.
- Pen, notepad or form
  - Make brief notes during the assessment, particularly of weights, to act as triggers when completing final documentation
- Stethoscope
  - For listening to swallowing

Before the mother or baby is touched, the mother should see the LC wash her hands for a full 30 second scrub with soap. Assessment includes palpation, visual assessment, and some auscultation. The physical and feeding assessment can be very detailed. For this monograph, a basic overview will be offered.

Maternal Assessment

The maternal assessment is at a basic level with the primary focus on the breast tissue and function. However, it is helpful to note some general things about the mother's appearance. If the mother is fully made up with hair styled, she may attach a lot of importance to her appearance. This is not necessarily wrong, but can certainly give a hint as to whether or not she is spending a lot of energy on personal and home appearance, rather than rest and sleep.

Edema

Mothers who have edema may also have trouble with milk expression as a result.

1. First observe the mother's face. Does it appear puffy? Is there periorbital edema (full swelling all around her eyes-not just bags underneath)? What does she have to say about her facial appearance-does it seem swollen to her? Mothers who have significant facial edema, most easily identified around the eyes, has some blood pressure trouble going on and will probably have breast tissue edema as well.

2. Next look at her hands. Ask her if she is able to wear her rings. If she can't, ask how long has it been since she last wore them?

3. Check her feet and ankles. It's easy to determine if the mother has pitting edema just by applying gentle pressure with a finger. If an indention remains, this is considered "pitting." Pitting edema is categorized as +1, +2, or +3 - the higher the level, the worse the edema.

4. Ask her if she feels like she is voiding or perspiring a lot. If not, normal postpartum diuresis (throwing off excess fluid volume needed during pregnancy) may not have occurred yet.

Some mothers with mild edema in their hands and feet still have significant edema in their chest wall or breast tissue. This is exacerbated by engorgement. A good way to determine this is to check for indention marks or skin ridges left by breast pads or the inner lining of a bra. The LC can perform reverse pressure softening to observe for fluid shift. This is a good teaching opportunity for the mother and will also be helpful if she is seen for latch difficulties (Cotterman, 2004).

Edema can be a sign of blood pressure problems, even if it was normal during pregnancy. If significant edema is observed, it may be a good idea to suggest that the mother talk to her physician about it, or the LC can send a copy of the consult notes to the OB.

Breast Assessment

Breast tissue should be assessed full on, in a side by side comparison. Noted should be size and shape, comparatively. While no mother has a complete bilateral match, average symmetry should exist. Significant bilateral variation in breast size or tissue fullness may indicate structural issues leading to potential supply challenges.

Breast size is unrelated to function, but certainly can relate to feeding difficulties. The mother with very large breasts and a small baby often has trouble seeing the baby at all, much less the latch. The mother with small breasts may have been taught breast support during latch, and as a result, her index finger is probably blocking the baby's chin, making deep latch impossible. Breasts that appear underdeveloped (not just small) can indicate insufficient glandular tissue.

The breast can be assessed in quadrants: the upper outer, upper inner, lower outer, and lower inner. This makes it easier to document blocked ducts or other tissue variations. In addition, if the assessment form has a line drawing to this effect, the LC can map the variations. Incision scars, moles, keloids, birthmarks, supernumerary tissue (the extra nipple a rare mom can have) and skin tags should also be described.

Skin should be assessed for color, tone, and feel. "Orange peel" skin is commonly found on fibrocystic breasts. If skin is red or tight, it should be palpated for engorgement, tenderness, or signs of infection. Note swelling and in instances where mastitis or abscess is suspected, it's helpful to outline the borders of the inflammation site in order to observe for an increase. Montgomery glands should be readily apparent, without signs of irritation or infection.

Nipple and Areola Assessment

Normal nipple surface should be rounded with even color pigmentation; flattening or inversion is important to note. If inverted, the mother should be asked to compare current state to pre-pregnancy state, as many inverted nipples will spontaneously evert. Inverted nipples are graded according to severity:

Grade 1- Nipple may be easily everted using a pump or other assistive device, or just by an effectively nursing baby.

Grade 2- Nipple may be everted, but will quickly invert before latch is obtained. This accounts for the majority of inverted nipples.

Grade 3- Nipple is impossible to evert.

Some fissures may be present, and the mother should be asked if they were present before breastfeeding. Unusually shaped or formed nipples, including size, should be described as clearly as possible. Nipple pores may be easily visible. The skin color of the areola should be evenly pigmented and may appear the same or darker than the skin on the nipple. The mother may also have hair on the areola or breast. The hair will not impact breastfeeding, although it can occasionally become infected.

Nipple trauma and pain are the most common reasons for early weaning. Trauma and pain should be assessed separately. Trauma can occur directly on the nipple or even on the areola. It can present as:

- abrasion
- blister
- scab
- crack
- rash
- bruise
- redness/irritation
- flaking

There may also be swelling, bleeding, pus if an infection is present, or a milk bleb as a blocked duct resolves. Skin color is important for identifying infection or inflammation, or even pain response. Baseline color should be established before a feeding, and then reassessed during and after a feed. Trauma will probably be present during a consultation for pain, but the LC should observe for additional trauma occurring during the feeding. The mother should be asked about self treatment for trauma because this may not come up during the history.

Pain

Pain assessment will be multilevel and will depend on what is being physically assessed. For example, the mother may be experiencing pain with engorgement, but also with feedings. This will need to be identified and documented separately because each pain response has a different care plan and represents a unique need for the mother, even though one may be related to the other. The pain assessment during the physical is pain the mother experiences at rest or between feedings.

Case Presentation Three - Trauma at an Inverted Nipple

This following case example shows how history is combined with assessment. Even using the limited information from the maternal history and assessment can give the LC direction for further observation and inquiry.

History-This mother was seen in her home at two weeks postpartum for a consultation relating to pain with feedings. She has an inverted nipple on the left side; the right side functions normally. She reported during the history that her nipple appeared to be somewhat everted during pregnancy, but never fully came out. She delivered by Cesarean section at term. In the hospital, latch on the left side was always painful. She was given a nipple shield, but states that it increased her pain, so she only used it once. She

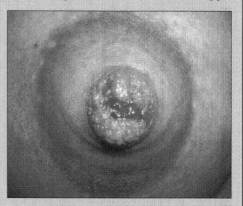

Recurrent nipple trauma

noticed abrading in the hospital, but then saw bleeding during feedings, and scabbing in between. She states that it now only hurts at the beginning and end of the feeding. She is using Lansinoh alone for the trauma.

Physical Assessment-The breast is full without engorgement or blocked ducts, areola soft. When the mother removed her breast pad, the scab had adhered to the material and tore away. Nipple assessment reveals that the center is still at least partially inverted. The trauma is in the shape of a compression stripe, centered at the inversion site, but continuing to the distal portion of the nipple.

Initial Impressions-In addition to the full baby physical and feeding assessments, the initial history and maternal assessment indicates several areas of special focus, or at least a need for additional information.
* The visual level of trauma indicates baby should be assessed for high or bubble palate and disorganized suck.

- The pain report indicates that trauma may not just be related to the inverted nipple. The baby may have been deep suctioned, since he was delivered by cesarean and should be assessed for clamping and oral aversion.
- In addition, the baby may be responding to a forceful MER; this should be a focused observation during the feeding assessment.
- With the inverted nipple and scabbing, the baby may have developed some "chewing" behaviors to allow for milk flow.
- Depending on suck issues, if the baby is swallowing a lot of air during the feeding, he may be clamping and arching when he feels gas pressure which would account for pain at the end of a feeding.

A common way to assess pain is to ask her to rate her pain using a scale, when she experiences it during the consultation. The rating is from 1-10, with one being mild pain and ten being the most extreme. Take the time to assess each type of pain variation the mother is experiencing.

Infant Assessment

Infant assessment can be quite lengthy; although generally speaking, a lactation consultant will only need to complete a fundamental assessment. The infant's basic appearance should be assessed to match developmental behaviors, physical appearance, and gestational age: a baby who was over 40 weeks at delivery should appear to be so developmentally. The LC will already be aware of due dates, delivery details, and whether the Dubowitz or Ballard score was completed. She will compare this to her observation and initial impression.

State

During the initial physical assessment before the feeding, the infant's state should be noted and the mother asked if it is typical, either before a feeding or for the majority of the day. For the mother of a baby who is barely a day old, this line of questioning is obviously deferred. Also noted should be the baby's response to intervention. If the baby is sleepy, is he easily roused or does it take full body massage and vestibulomotor stimulation? If the baby is fussy, note how long and what it takes to calm him (swaddling, sucking, the father comforting, and so on). As the LC is gathering her first impressions of the baby's state, she should observe his environment.

> *Teaching Tip: The very newborn state is hugely affected by environment, as well as medical condition. In the hospital, many new parents are proud of their new baby who is already sleeping so well. The ILC can discuss how sleep states shut out excessive stimulation. The ILC can also prepare parents for the first few nights at home in a quieter environment.*

Skin

The baby's skin should be assessed in general. If the baby is jaundiced, has a rash, or has skin break-down, a full body assessment is then necessary. With jaundice in particular, further description is helpful:

- Where-face, sclera, trunk, full body
- How much-descriptive terms, accompanied by recent blood levels if available
- Current treatment-sun, phototherapy, supplemental feeds
- Maximum severity-hospitalization, highest levels

Normal infant acne, cradle cap, or even eczema may not be important unless ruling out a food sensitivity or allergy.

Head, Neck and Shoulders

If the birth was assisted by forceps or vacuum, molding and caput (swelling and bruising on baby's head) should be noted. The extent of any bruising is important, as it can directly relate to newborn jaundice. Assisted births or intrauterine positioning during late pregnancy can often lead to some facial asymmetry, potentially creating latch and positioning difficulties. The side of the asymmetry and amount should be stated (mild, moderate) in descriptive terms. Ask the mother if the infant tends to hold, turn, or drop his head to one side. If present, the LC can feel along the infant's neck muscles for signs of torticollis. Head, neck, shoulders, and upper body in general should be in basic alignment when the infant is at rest.

Even the very newborn will raise his head for brief intervals when awake, and the older infant will hold his head up for longer periods of time. The shape of the head is important to note, molding will be present when a vaginal birth occurs, little to none with a cesarean section-depending on whether the mother labored. Some skull flattening may be present if the baby spends long periods of time on his back. This condition has significantly increased since the Back to Sleep SIDS campaign (Persing et al., 2003).

Oral Cavity and Suck

The infant's mouth should be visually assessed: looking for color variations, palate formation, gum line, and tongue shape and movement. If the tongue appears coated, it should be gently wiped with gauze to rule out thrush. Typically, a visual observation occurs when an infant is crying or yawning and the mouth is in a wide gape. Often, it is helpful to complete a visual assessment during a diaper change.

Using a clean, gloved finger with short nails, digital assessment should be gentle and completed in a minimal amount of time. Too long of a digital assessment can be a form of suck training and impact a feeding observation. LCs should follow basic rules for latch by stroking the infant's lips to stimulate rooting and only inserting the gloved finger with a wide gape, rather than forcing it in. An index finger is probably ideal for palpation assessment, since sensitivity is greater. The finger should be pad down to assess tongue positioning, movement, and mobility, then rotate upward to feel the palate formation and ridges. The LC should document how the palate looks and feels-high palate, flattened, bubble, and so on.

Suck organization is a collaboration of mouth/lip seal without compression, tongue movement in a wavelike motion with full extension over gum, pulling sensation with vacuum, relaxed jaw, and intermittent swallowing of saliva. Variation of an organized suck can include but is not limited to: vacuum without movement, tight jaw, lip compression-upper, lower or both, or chewing motions with a retracted or fluttering tongue. Guarding or self protective behaviors are commonly found in babies with oral trauma, such as deep or vigorous suctioning.

> *Teaching Opportunity: As the LC progresses through the baby assessment, she should tell the family what she is observing and what she is looking for. It is reassuring to parents when they are told that their baby is developmentally appropriate, especially when this is clearly defined. Often, the LC is there because things are going wrong-pointing out the positives is encouraging for the mother.*

Chapter Six

FEEDING ASSESSMENT

The mother should be encouraged to demonstrate feeding and latch techniques that she is already using. If the LC begins a feeding assessment with instruction, not only will this not allow her to accurately identify where problems may be occurring, but can actually create feeding difficulties. The mother may also have undermined confidence, believing that she can't do anything right, since changes in the feeding are occurring before the assessment really starts.

Intake Weights

In the outpatient or private practice settings, intake weights should be completed as part of the feeding assessment. This is generally started when the baby is at least three days old. The scale must be digital and accurate within two grams (Cadwell et al., 2006), although it doesn't have to be made by a specific manufacturer. For an intake weight, it also isn't necessary for a baby to be unclothed; it may be better for the feeding if he is dressed, since this can over-stimulate many babies, making latch more difficult. The LC should note all weights, rather than rely on a memory feature on the scale. If a diaper absolutely must be changed mid-feeding, intake should be fully calculated before a reweigh.

If the baby's overall growth weights are questionable, the LC should obtain an accurate total baby weight at the end of the consultation when the baby is calm. This can be done with the baby either unclothed or with a fresh, dry diaper only. The LC should specify which way the baby was weighed in her documentation.

Positioning

The LC should note how the mother is holding and supporting both her baby and her breast. First time mothers may be afraid of the baby's head, particularly the soft spot areas. She should be asked why she is using a particular position or technique-is it more comfortable for her? Mothers closely study books and website images and may be trying to "match the picture." Pillows, according to type and how they are used, should be briefly listed, and the mother should be asked if they are used for every feeding or a majority of feedings.

How or if a mother supports her breast should be documented. If the mother is using assistive devices for large or pendulous breasts, the LC should list the type and whether the devise is used for every or a majority of feedings.

Latch

All of the elements of latch, from hunger cues to visible swallowing of colostrum to audible swallows indicating milk transfer, should be carefully detailed - whether present or not. Allowing the mother to obtain the latch herself if possible, even if it appears incorrect, will not only help the LC with problem identification, but establish the mother's knowledge base. If the mother is having difficulty obtaining a latch, the LC should help only one step at a time, allowing the mother and baby an opportunity to progress on their own.

If the baby is sleeping, the mother should rouse the baby when typical hunger cues (rooting, smacking, tongue thrusting) are exhibited, using her own instinctive or learned techniques. The mother should be encouraged to trigger or stimulate several hunger cues before attempting to latch, particularly in the inpatient setting where babies will often fall asleep with a too early latch attempt.

Once feeding readiness is indicated by the baby, the mother then progresses through the elements of latch while the LC observes (in general):
• Stimulates rooting to the gape
  - Brushes the nipple on the lip, rests the nipple on the philtrum, or hand expresses colostrum for smacking and licking
  - Baby turns or roots to nipple
• Pulls baby in
  -Supports baby, brings baby to mother instead of the reverse
  -Baby's head and body are aligned
  -Mother sits back rather than leans forward, shoulders appear relaxed
• Latch-on
  - Baby's mouth/jaw is wide open, lip line is visible, chin doubled, nares clear/flared
  - If LC can pull lower lip back, baby's tongue over gum line, cupping nipple
  - Baby's cheeks rounded and smooth
  - Nipple deep in baby's mouth
  - Head may be slightly tilted
  - Mother has no pain
• Suck pattern
  - Sucking active; rate is rapid, even paced, slow, or intermittent

- Rhythm self sustained or needs stimulation
- Accessory muscle contracture visible (temple, jaw hinge, ears)
- Movement smooth and gliding rather than jagged
- Note sounds of suction break, such as clicks or squeaks
• Swallows
- With colostrum, swallowing subtle and primarily visible. This can be auscultated with a stethoscope, but this is likely to disrupt a feeding and suggest medical necessity to the mother; use only when necessary.
- Transitional or mature milk has larger volumes, swallowing audible and visible
• Release
- At end of feeding or when needing to burp, baby slips off breast
- Note clamping or non-nutritive sucking, and if the end of the feeding is mother guided

The baby's behavior throughout the feeding should always be noted. In particular, the baby should be observed for stimulation sucks, how he copes with let-down, and how the feeding is paused for burping. If any assistive devices, such as a nipple shield or Mini SNS, are used, the mother should be able to articulate how they are used, as well as demonstrate their use; although, the initial feeding attempt should be without assistive devices. Finally, infant behavior and suck pattern at the end of the feeding and how the feeding is finished should be noted, in addition to burp techniques - ease and effectiveness.

If there is a variation from the norm at any time during the latch process and the LC has made her assessment, she can then instruct the mother and make any corrections needed to improve the latch before continuing to the next step. Changes are generally documented as part of the intervention or plan, even though this may seem out of context when applied to the assessment.

Pain

When pain occurs during the feeding, it becomes a separate entity from other pain assessments. Even if the LC has already documented that the mother feels pain in her nipple, the pain may be only one element of a multi-dimensional problem. Having the mother describe her pain sensations during or immediately after a feeding will provide more key details for solving feeding issues. Pain may be general, but it is more often specific to certain conditions or issues.

Suggesting descriptive terminology, such as pinching, rubbing, or burning, will help her articulate more precisely something that can be very difficult to describe. She should also be asked to identify what makes the pain better or worse and whether it is always the same intensity. It is important to reassure her to report even brief pain or mild tenderness, since many mothers think (or are told) that some pain is a normal part of breastfeeding.

The pain report should always be compared with the history, physical assessment, and feeding assessment to establish an accurate cause or causes.

Case Presentation Four: The Balance of History and Assessment

Mrs. A scheduled a consult for pain and nipple trauma and to rule out yeast.

Significant History

Mrs. A is a first time mother, far from home and family, with support from her husband, who was only able to take one week off work. Her cultural background is different from the U.S.; in her country, breastfeeding is the norm, as is female family assistance for several weeks after delivery. She is very anxious to parent correctly and also has concerns about the well-being of her baby. She works in healthcare and admits that fear of potential problems that she sees in her work add to her anxiety level.

Her nipple trauma first occurred in the hospital within the first few feedings. She was briefly visited by an LC, but a feeding was not observed. She was given a nipple shield for pain, but this increased her trauma, so she stopped using it after discharge.

She was treated with antibiotics for a urinary tract infection for five days.

She contacted her obstetrician and also spoke with an outpatient LC at three weeks postpartum for continued trauma, pain, and burning in between and during feedings. At this time, she was prescribed Difflucan for two weeks; the baby was treated prophylactically with Nystatin swabs. She states that her pain did not change or improve during or after treatment. As a result, she scheduled a home visit with a PPLC.

Significant Assessment

The baby's mouth was clear, with no signs of thrush. The oral assessment revealed a bubble palate and suck callus at the upper lip, with some initial clamping and lip compression. No signs of tongue tie.

- Back to history for possible cause of clamping-mother delivered with vacuum assist. States no deep suctioning that she is aware of.

Appearance and developmental behaviors, in addition to suck, appears near rather than full term.

- History reveals mother had elective induction at 38 weeks.
- Long epidural; approximately 10 hours.

Visual assessment reveals that nipple tip has circular open wound; probably rubbing in bubble palate space.

Significant Feeding Assessment

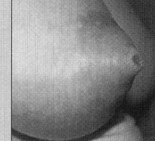

No pain before this feeding. However, mother felt pain with initial latch, observed shallow latch with upper lip compression. Pain improved with asymmetrical latch techniques and deeper latch obtained.

Observed non-nutritive suck when baby started to fall asleep, but Mrs. A can feel the difference in suck and will break latch. No pain with non-nutritive suck.

Nipple assessment - before a feeding with trauma

Mrs. A states she typically airs nipple after feeding, then replaces her bra. Approximately 4-5 minutes after feeding, while discussing the feeding plan, she felt burning and pain in her nipple. Bra removed for reassessment.

Physical Reassessment

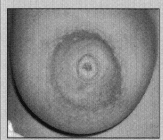

Blanching is beyond the nipple into the areola. Duration is about one minute, then color changes to red and back to pink.

- Additional history needed-mother states she "always has cold hands and feet." In addition, she is susceptible to cold sensations in winter or even at the grocery store where frozen foods are stored. She recalls feeling nipple pain after showering, but thought it was related to infection.

Same breast, approximately 5 minutes after a feeding with blanching related to vasospasm.

Mrs. A's primary pain is related to repeated nipple trauma, with secondary pain from vasospasm. She may also have Raynaud's Disease based on her history of cold response, although this is a medical condition to be determined by her primary caregiver. As a result, a copy of the consult findings should be sent to the OB as well as the Ped for continuity of care.

> *Teaching Opportunity: Because pain with breastfeeding is such a commonly held myth, this is the time to teach the mother otherwise. The LC can explain what she is looking for in terms of a good latch, as well as pain responses. When correcting the latch, the LC should endeavor to explain why a specific pattern behavior, such as lip compression, is painful.*

After the Feeding

The baby's behavior, after feeding at the breast appears complete, is very important. Once again, the mother should be encouraged to compare the current behavior to other observed behaviors after feedings. The time of actual nutritive sucking should be noted to create a "snap shot in time," with the understanding that the length of feedings will continue to vary, along with actual intake.

How the mother feels about the feeding is of primary importance. The LC may think everything is perfect, but unless the mother agrees, problems will continue.

Supplement

If supplement has been ongoing, this feeding should be observed as well. For the outpatient or PPLC, quite often the baby has been supplemented by bottle with expressed breast milk or formula. If so, the LC should initiate the bottle feed to observe how well the baby tolerates the milk flow, nipple, and method of feeding in general. She should observe the mother or support person feeding the baby in order to address any technique issues.

If supplement is given by cup or syringe, the mother should demonstrate use if she is already familiar with the technique. If the tool is new, the LC will first offer instruction, then observe the mother demonstrating the technique (return demonstration).

> *Teaching Tip: Paced bottle feedings, also referred to as the Kassing Method, are an excellent way to help parents identify subtle feeding cues and avoid overfeeding. Because the feeding is at a slower rate, the baby will take in less air while having his sucking need better met. This is a technique that can be easily taught, even to older siblings, with very positive outcomes (Attachment F).*

Pumping

Quite often, if a mother is having feeding difficulties and a pump hasn't been introduced already, it needs to be introduced during the consult. If the mother already has a pump, she should be asked to demonstrate its use. The

LC should document the pump type and brand, as well as whether it is new or previously used. If she doesn't have a pump, the LC should have access to one to at least demonstrate effective technique, with the mother providing a return demonstration to get her started in a routine, if indicated.

Introduction of a pump is only necessary if the baby is unable to transfer milk efficiently, the baby is unable to stimulate lactogenesis alone, or the mother specifically requests assistance with pumping.

Attachment F

The Kassing Method for Paced Bottle Feeding

BOTTLE-FEEDING THE BREASTFED BABY
Dee Kassing, BS, MLS, IBCLC, RLC

1. Use straight bottle, not bent.

2. Use bottle with small-mouthed opening, not a disposable or wide-mouthed bottle.

3. Nipple should have an old-fashioned long, round shape. The base of the nipple should be about 1 inch (25 mm) across, and the base should preferably be tapered, not bulbous. The nipple should **not** be orthodontic, stubby, or shaped like a miniature human breast.

4. Nipple should be a slow-flow nipple, unless otherwise directed by the lactation consultant.

5. Support baby in an upright position. Babies younger than two months will usually need support for the lower back. This can be accomplished by the caregiver crossing her/his legs and setting the baby on the lower leg with back against higher leg. Or, the caregiver can place one foot on a footstool. If sitting in a chair with high arms, a pillow can be tucked against baby's back. Caregiver can support baby's head and neck by placing the thumb behind one of the baby's ears and fingers behind the other ear. Hold head firmly enough to keep baby's chin up off chest.

6. Gently brush nipple DOWN over center of baby's lips. Pull nipple away from face and center nipple in front of baby's mouth. Pause. Wait for baby to open WIDE, like a yawn. If baby does not open WIDE after pausing, caregiver may repeat downward stroke of nipple. If baby still does not open WIDE, try gently tapping nipple two to three times on baby's lower lip. Pull nipple away from face and center nipple in front of baby's mouth. When baby opens WIDE, insert nipple all the way into mouth, so baby's lips touch the collar that holds the nipple onto the bottle.

7. Tip up bottom of bottle just enough so milk covers the hole in the nipple. (Healthy full term babies will pause and breathe on their own. If you are working with a young premie or a neurologically impaired baby, you may have to periodically tip the bottle so no milk remains in the nipple to allow the baby to pause and breathe.)

8. When there is very little food left in the bottle, lean baby's body back about 45 degrees. This will keep his head and neck in line, yet allow the bottle to tip for remainder of feeding.

Bottle-feeding baby in this manner should take approximately 15-20 minutes. If feedings consistently take 30 minutes or longer, please contact your lactation consultant (Kassing, 2002).

Chapter Seven

UNIQUE SITUATIONS

This chapter consists of atypical history and physical assessment findings or uncommon family situations. The topics included may be rare, occasional, or growing. There is very little information on many of these topics in current resources.

Even the most seasoned LC can be perplexed about how to get a baby latched around a nipple ring. Rare is the LC who is comfortable assessing a mother for signs of abuse. However, because all of these topics relate to breastfeeding support, the LC has a responsibility to be knowledgeable about these issues.

Piercing

The current generation of mothers has embraced body art as a means of self expression, as well as a fashion statement - most commonly tattooing and piercing. While existing tattoos generally do not impact breastfeeding, nipple piercing might. The presence of piercing does not create a contraindication for breastfeeding, but rather it requires further history and assessment (Martin, 2004).

History taking for a mother who has a piercing will include the specifics of the procedure, especially when it was done and if it was performed by a piercing professional versus a friend. The mother should be asked about the healing process and whether there were any difficulties or infection. Other good questions to ask are whether the mother removes her jewelry, if she has any trouble replacing it, and if there is any discharge from the site.

Physical examination will include assessment for scarring, keloids, or discoloration of the skin. The site should be palpated for knotty tissue/blocked ducts and leaking. During palpation, as well as during the feeding, the mother should be questioned about decreased sensitivity or numbness. Conversely, some mothers report increased sensitivity, particularly with jewelry in place.

Nipple piercing can take a long time to heal: anywhere from eight to twelve months. After this time, it is generally considered safe to remove jewelry. Jewelry should be removed for the safety of the baby, as well as to avoid impairing the latch and suck. Although some of the current lactation related literature suggests that mothers can use temporary jewelry to keep the piercing open, the Association of Professional Piercers recommends that no jewelry be present during feedings. The piercing can rapidly close during a feeding, even if the opening was made several years ago. The mother can contact her piercer to check or reopen the site with an insertion taper, but most will recommend that she have it repierced after weaning. Obtaining a new nipple piercing during lactation is contraindicated, and the APP recommends waiting at least three months after milk production stops to repierce.

After feeding at a piercing site, intake should be assessed and the breast palpated for full or blocked ducts if scarring is present.

Abuse

Intimate partner abuse is currently a term that can mean either physical or emotional abuse. According to a study in JOGNN, abuse occurs during pregnancy, with average rates of 3.9-8.3% (Lutz, 2005). The number of abused women who go on to breastfeed is unknown, but it can be assumed that some will. For the LC, this can be difficult to identify. This issue creates discomfort for many healthcare providers, and the mother may have never been asked about abuse. Screening for suspected, ongoing abuse should be more than checking a box. It may be helpful to include a reassurance statement, then ask an open-ended question about the abuse the mother may have experienced.

Example: A reassurance statement may be: "Because we have learned that partner abuse is more common than most people realize, part of the history taking includes asking you about this…", followed by a direct, open-ended question.

The ILC should be aware of organizational policy when abuse is identified. She will most likely have to contact an in-house medical social worker or a case manager, who will then follow up with a further needs assessment and assistance. The PPLC is more isolated, and as a result, should be aware of mandatory reporting guidelines and community resources for the mother.

Mothers should be screened for past sexual abuse. In some cases, this type of abuse can cause feeding and possibly pumping difficulties. The mother who was abused may be ambivalent, revolted, or empowered about breastfeeding - there isn't a predictable response. If breastfeeding or the idea of breastfeeding seems to be causing a resurgence of past fears or trauma, the LC should help the mother find a mental health professional for further assistance. Cynthia Good Mojab is a Lactational Psychologist (LC and mental health professional) who created an excellent dialogue/script style essay that may assist LCs to find the right words in this situation (Attachment G). The LC should continue to assess breastfeeding or breastmilk feeding needs to provide additional support.

The NICU Baby

Babies are admitted to the intensive care unit for a variety of reasons. The length of stay can vary greatly and is dependent on the baby's age and medical condition. A term or near-term baby may be in the NICU to rule out sepsis, or they may have transient tachypnea of the newborn (TTN). Both conditions require a stay of one week or less. Others infants may have more complex conditions, such as respiratory distress requiring oxygen. Some are called "feeder-growers." They are generally born at 32-37 weeks gestation and will only need to reach a specific weight and tolerate feedings by mouth before they are discharged. The most fragile are very low birth weight (VLBW) babies, born less than 32 weeks and/or 1500 grams, and the babies with anomalies and/or who require surgery. These very critical babies average a NICU stay of two to three months, but can easily stay longer.

A baby who has spent any time in the NICU can present with breastfeeding challenges as a result. While the baby is still hospitalized, the ILC will probably be mostly focused on assisting the mother will supply issues and pumping. She needs to be aware of maternal fatigue, slower medical recovery, and the impact of stress on the mother's milk supply. She may help transition the baby to breast, but often, depending on the environment, this is one of the last steps before discharge.

After discharge, the outpatient or PPLC may assist the dyad with transitioning to breast, weaning from supplement, weight gain, or weaning from assistive devices. This may be attempted while the mother is also juggling medical appointments, treatments, and care of a baby who may still have health issues. Regardless of the practice setting, there is specific information that should be obtained that is unique to these babies.

As part of the history, the LC should ascertain how much time the mother has spent at the hospital with the baby (Gonzales et al., 2003). Research has shown that the more time and involvement the mother has with the care of the baby, the better the transition from NICU to home. Involvement includes gaining familiarity with the monitors, participating in daily care needs if possible, touching and stroking the baby, kangaroo care, and interacting with hospital staff.

Ideally, an actively involved mother is there at least every day for more than one feeding. To obtain this information, the LC can interview the mother, but should be cautious to avoid sounding judgmental or critical - regardless of the mother's interaction level. The LC can get input from the NICU staff, either from shift report or one on one. The mother should be questioned regarding knowledge and whether she attends specific support groups, either for NICU parents or breastfeeding, in addition to any related postpartum classes.

Once the baby is discharged, history should include rationale (such as additional protein) for supplemental feeds and how long they will be necessary, medical equipment in use, other care providers involved for additional medical needs, and daily or weekly travel for care. Many mothers feel obligated to continue the feeding and care schedules initiated in the hospital and discussion of this should be solicited.

Assessment of the mother will include an observation of displayed confidence or comfort level handling medical equipment, as well as how she handles the baby. Along with the basic assessment, the baby will also be observed for oral aversion, sensitivity to light and noise levels, touch, and over-stimulation. Because the intensive care environment is loud and busy, many babies who have spent a long time there do not respond well to quiet. Babies who have had many IVs and blood draws may strongly react when their feet are touched. Though atypical for an average newborn, the LC should be aware that these behaviors are expected with these babies.

Most of these mothers and babies will need follow up, since their challenges are likely to be greater and their progression steps smaller. Ongoing assessment should be focused on maternal fatigue and stress and infant overload.

Multiples

An informal survey was sent to an email list of a local affiliate for the National Mothers of Multiples Club. The mothers were asked to share their biggest challenges, breastfeeding and otherwise, when caring for more than one newborn. They were also asked what they felt healthcare professionals should know about mothers of multiples, and how they could be best supported.

The majority of responses occurred in the first three hours after the initial email was sent. Most were very detailed: some were humorous, others were heart-wrenching. Most included a telephone number in case further information was needed. Because their comments go beyond what research can show, a sampling has been included - edited only for grammar, spelling, or repeated content.

I quickly remember the frustrations I had with nursing twins… aaahh! After talking to 4 different lactations consultants, the most frustrating part for me was they didn't seem to "get it" that it was different for us, making me feel even dumber. I did "ok" until about 6 weeks, when they were starting to move around and I could no longer nurse them at the same time…which meant 45 min. at the minimum to feed, when I was still feeding every 3 hours. Also, they had me pumping after each time I nursed, which meant another 10+minutes to pump, as well as clean equipment, get babies cared for, etc…then it was time to do it all over again. I will never forget one consultant told me I needed to "accept the fact that all I was going to do some days was sit on the couch and nurse"… which may have been ok at 2 weeks, but by 6 weeks, you're ready to do something else sometimes. I pushed through to 5 months, but I must say the whole experience was miserable and purely out of obligation (I also had mastitis 2 times). I also was unable to produce enough milk, so they ended up nursing every other feeding…one nursed and one bottle fed each time. The consultants continued to say I would produce more milk if I pumped after each feeding, but I just did not find it to work in my situation. I'm still puzzled by the whole experience. Had my MD not been so adamant I push through, I probably would have given up very early on. I'm very hopeful for a totally different experience with one child!
-Kristy

I remember the most difficult thing for me (other than postpartum depression!) was feeding. I was scheduling the babies and wanted to feed them at the same time. Trying to give bottles to 4-pound, sleepy preemies in bouncy seats (in the middle of the night!) is tough for one person. I would prop their necks up so that they could take the bottle without me having to hold them. Another huge issue for me at birth was breastfeeding in the NICU and worrying about how much they were getting. I decided to pump so that I knew exactly how much they were taking in.
-Kelly

For me it was being so overwhelmed with two preemies being discharged at the same time with numerous follow-up appointments, such as pediatrician, ophthalmologist, pulmonologist, and etcetera. We had a home health nurse coming several times a week for weight checks. We had the apnea monitors to deal with. So in addition to being terribly sleep deprived, I was overwhelmed with healthcare professionals (of which I am one and my husband is a physician). I must confess I was unable to breastfeed as I had no milk after 4 weeks of pumping while mine were in the NICU.
-Jeannie

When my twins were born, I was sick. I really wanted to nurse and had been told by lactation consultants to give my boys only breastmilk. I was trying very hard. The pediatrician finally told me that my boys needed more nutrition. She told me to nurse, then give them some formula. If she hadn't told me to do that, I probably would have felt like a failure and given up on nursing. I think it is important for new moms to know that breastmilk is best, but there are options when you have a low milk supply. I also believe pumping (especially with multiples or sick moms) is not the only way to increase milk supply. As a result of the support I received, I nursed my twins until 13 months. If I had not been told that a formula/breastmilk combination was an option, I probably would have given up.
-Margaret

I was a first time Mom with my twins and breastfeeding them exclusively, not counting the sleep deprivation, I had really excruciatingly sore nipples (I felt like I had been dragged across a gravel driveway topless) due to my twins really wanting to nurse often and my daughter's latch on was a clamping down Nightmare, she didn't have a good latch on. Nothing really helped but cream and time or calluses formed, not sure. I also had a rash called PUPPS spread all over my arms, legs, and stomach (Really Itchy) 1st weeks were quite miserable. I was a wreck - so glad I didn't have postpartum depression too.
-Meghan

My biggest problem trying to nurse my preemie triplets, I was huge compared to a 3 pound baby. I couldn't hold them the traditional way; I could only do the football hold. Their faces were so tiny that it seemed like they were smothered.

-Brenda

My B/G twins were born at 33 weeks and had to learn to eat, regulate body temp, and completely breathe on their own. Other than that, they were very healthy. Both lost weight during their stay, and I constantly worried about their weight and feedings; how much and how long it took them because every calorie counted. They were unable to breastfeed, so I pumped for them, and the most success I had at that was right there in the NICU, just being with them. I rented a pump and kept it crib side and had a portable one for me at home and traveling. I would always produce the most milk when I was with them. It was amazing. The nurses pulled the curtain for privacy, would tell the LC when I was there for convenient help.

One HUGE difference I could tell in my babies overall comfort was keeping them in the same bassinet vs. separate. They snuggled, slept better, and seemed to eat better by staying awake more during feedings and taking in more. This eating benefit was obvious after the NG tube came out and I was feeding them. I use to get so upset when I would walk into the NICU and they were separated. I later learned that there were a handful of nurses who were not comfortable with putting them together. I made sure this was changed when it came to my babies but that seems like an education opportunity for the hospital and the staff.

My twins just turned 3 and some of this feels as fresh as yesterday.

-Shannon

I would emphasize the importance of learning how to feed them both at the same time ALONE. Learning how to get my boys in a comfortable position by myself was a huge challenge for me.

-Christa

The one thing that bothered me a lot was nurses and lactation consultants that thought they were helping but kept saying over and over again that it should not be painful. I was a new mom learning to nurse and nursing twins my breasts never got to rest. It was very painful for the first week or so until my nipples got used to it and my babies got used to it. I hated that no one realized that not having down time for either nipple though really could be more painful and difficult.

-Jenny

My twins were born at 32 weeks but I was hospitalized 2 weeks prior (after 10 weeks bedrest at home). While in the high risk unit, I was treated like a queen!!! After their births I was sent off to some floor while the babies were in NICU of course. My recovery was slow, I didn't get to even see them for 26 hours. My problem lies with post partum. Since I was not bringing the babies into my room (nor did I see any in the area I was in), I kinda got neglected. In fact, a lactation nurse finally CALLED me after many requests to the nurse about pumping. Equipment was sent with very little instructions. Because they were early, it was even harder to get milk flowing, especially after a good 2 days went by before I began pumping. I just feel like if my babies had been with me and were going to truly nurse from me that I would have gotten better 'treatment' (for lack of a better word).

-Angie

Assisting mothers of multiples present unique challenges for the LC in any setting. The biggest difficulty that these mothers encounter is the fact that they are treated the same as mothers of singletons, leading to much frustration for them since their problems are not the same. The complications of pregnancy alone can lead to breastfeeding issues, so the LC should be aware of challenges within this population.

Pregnancy and birth complications for the mother can include:
- Hypertension, preeclampsia, or HELLP syndrome
- Anemia
- Preterm labor
- Perinatal bleeding or hemorrhage

- Gestational diabetes
- Bedrest-related complications, such as muscular deterioration and loss of stamina
- Difficulty with bonding and attachment

From a statistical standpoint, twins or higher order multiples (HOM) are significantly more at risk to be delivered very preterm (32 weeks or less). Singletons have a risk of 2%, twins 14%, and triplets 40% (Damato et al., 2005). It is much more likely that multiples, especially HOM, will be spending some time in the NICU. Additional complications for the babies are:

- Low birth weight or intrauterine growth retardation (IUGR)
- Discordant growth
- Twin to twin transfusion syndrome
- Increased risk of congenital anomalies
- Increased risk of surgery
- Increased risk of fetal death

Maternal and infant medical complications can thread into greater breastfeeding issues, including:

- Insufficient milk production
- Painful feedings
- Mastitis due to inefficient emptying
- Yeast due to trauma or antibiotic use
- Poor weight gain
- Disorganized suck

All of these complications, the physical, emotional and financial challenges or medical complications of multiples, can put the mother at greater risk for postpartum depression-as much as two to three times higher. As a result, the history should be more detailed in terms of the pregnancy, as well as the birth. The ILC may spend more time teaching and less time on feeding assessment if the babies are in the NICU setting. However, the outpatient or PPLC will focus more on the babies' history from birth to the current setting, particularly the feeding history. Each baby should have an individualized history. Determining unique differences between each baby will be difficult for the LC, making the interview in this situation even more important. Additional information for the history will include pumping practices, maternal education, and maternal knowledge base.

Whether the mother feeds both babies together or separately depends on the mother's preference. Mothers are often told to feed their babies together, but not all are able, or even want, to do this. If she can't feed simultaneously, then the assessment can be a teaching opportunity as well, but this will greatly depend on the family; this can't be forced. If feeding together, it may be better for the LC to observe each baby latch several times in order to better differentiate feeding patterns. Often when fed together, the baby with the weaker suck may not latch well or only demonstrate non-nutrative sucking until the stronger baby triggers the MER. Assistive feeding devices and other breastfeeding equipment will probably be in place. The mother's knowledge and demonstrated use should be assessed as well.

Additional consultations will probably be necessary simply because the babies will learn and develop at different rates. This may benefit the mother who is probably taking in less information because she is stressed.

Adoption

Adopting mothers have very unique, individualized needs. The adopting mother's first point of contact with an LC may be during the adoption process, when she is seeking information or care for inducing lactation. Conversely, she may show up at the hospital after the birth mother has delivered and may or may not be already working with an LC. Regardless, because of the complexity of adoption, the LC will need to allocate more time for the adopting mother's history, as well as communicating with her and her support system.

If a history form is used to support an adopting mother, information about the adoption should be listed. This will be fluid, depending on the situation. Making a form "fit" a mother may be impossible, particularly when inducing lactation, so the LC in any setting will probably want to use S.O. A. P. charting or some other narrative format.

Demographic information to include (as much as possible) will be names and contact information for the adopting mother's attorney, social worker, and involved healthcare providers, such as a family practitioner, gynecologist, and pediatrician. If the adoption is open, details can be obtained regarding the birth mother's general health, pregnancy history, and prenatal care. The adopting mother's health history should be explored in greater detail, particularly her reproductive history (onset of menses, breast development, and pregnancy history). If the birth hospital is identified, it is a good idea for an outpatient or PPLC to obtain permission to communicate with the ILC to facilitate breastfeeding or pumping when the baby is born - a sort of "inside connection." The ILC can serve as a bridge after delivery for other organizational resources, such as nursing, case management or social work, and even hospital supervisors who can assist with locating an empty room for the adopting mother to feed, pump, or even stay in.

Finally, the adoptive mother's knowledge base regarding induced lactation, as well as a frank discussion of plan adjustment if the adoption falls through is critical. Induced lactation is a huge commitment on all levels (including that of the LC), so all involved should have a clear understanding of each step in the process.

Assessment will probably begin with return demonstration of care and use of a pump. If the baby arrives before any artificial stimulation occurs, a first breastfeeding assessment will preclude any equipment use, since a nursing baby is the best stimulation. Other equipment needs can include an SNS, Lact-Aid, Finger Feeder, shields, or shells. Their use should be determined on an individualized basis after history and assessment. The use of these items will be part of the plan, as well as reassessment.

Example: An example of an outpatient consultation reveals that with adoption, a significant portion of the consult is the history, followed by knowledge assessment and planning. Because there are multiple communication factors, documentation is a combination of a systems review or a look at the mother's overall health within each body system that can potentially impact breastfeeding and narrative charting because results are so variable that a form would be incomplete.

Case Presentation Five-History and Assessment for Prenatal Consultation

<u>Outpatient Consult</u>   <u>1/2/06, 1400</u>
Ann Adopting (DOB 7/28/70)   **Husband/Frank**
123 Street, Columbia, SC 29999
Home: 888-8888   Cell: 111-1111   Email: personal email@aol.com

Gyn: Dr. Smith (Michelle, RN) 222-2222
Ped: Dr. Jones/Big Ped Group 333-3333
Attorney: Jay Harris, JD/Big Law Firm 444-4444
Birth Mother: Jane Birth

Initially contacted by pt by email one week ago for information regarding lactation services; self-referred via ILCA, Medela (web search). Discussed pros and cons for pt consideration, website resources given. Pt called back and scheduled prenatal consult for today. Medical history is verbal and written per pt; see attached. **(Author's note: Many women with a long history of fertility problems become accustomed to keeping a summary of their medical history. It is good idea to ask about this summary when setting up the appointment time. A copy can be reviewed and placed with the record, saving the LC a lot of time.)**

<u>Current Meds</u>-Folic Acid/B vitamin supplement, Synthroid 0.75 mcg

<u>Allergies</u>-PCN

<u>Diet/Herbals</u>: no specific diet needs or preferences. No herbal therapies/ natural remedies or teas.

<u>Social:</u> Pt is 35 y.o. MWF who is employed as a software designer (part time). Husband is currently working in sales. Adopted son at birth (4/20/04); open adoption, still maintaining written contact with birth mother. Did not know about induced lactation with first child. Extended family is out of state; has lived in Columbia one year.

<u>Reproductive:</u> Pt is multigravida of unknown number-many losses less than 12 weeks relating to implantation failure. Has had full fertility workup with exp. lap. No variations in hormone levels per workup notes.

Onset of menses age 13, states normal breast development starting age 10. Has taken birth control pills in past without difficulty; none at this time.

Other Medical: Hypothyroid well managed by Synthroid. Hx of depression; no longer needing meds. Has taken Zoloft in the past.

Surgical -Multiple laparoscopies, partial removal of ovary ('01).

Adoption Details -Began private domestic adoption process about six months ago; contacted by lawyer last month for match. Birth mother is currently incarcerated at Named Correctional Facility. EDC is March 30; arrested in July, sentenced in August when pregnancy was discovered. Pt knows birth mother had some drug use, probably smoking crack but arrest was unrelated. Birth mother has had prenatal care since August, pt reports pregnancy uncomplicated. Pt reports birth mother has two other children in foster care who have bonded and will remain with caregivers. Adoption is open, pt and birth mother communicate at least once a week. Pt states that birth mother seems very positive about decision making and pt feels comfortable with process. Induction date is March 20 for term delivery.

Plan: Pt has already reviewed Newman protocols. Prefers to start the accelerated protocol, modified, for at least 30 days; longer is preferable. With MD approval, will start with birth control only, then switch to galactagogues and stimulation when med is d/c'd. Reglan undesirable r/t pt Hx of depression, will consider Domperidone. Discussed common herbal galactagogues (Fenugreek, More Milk Plus). Pt is willing to try Fenugreek with pumping. Pt to discuss decisions regarding herbal and medication supplements with Dr Smith before proceeding. Will begin pumping with hospital grade double electric pump on daily regime when BCP stops. If baby comes early, pt will d/c BCP and will attempt to supplement at breast with SNS for stimulation. Pt will discuss BF with birth mother to obtain permission to feed before paperwork completed. Plan for f/u with home visit after adoption to assess intake or any feeding difficulties. I will contact hospital LC, and fax notes. Pt verbalized understanding of and agreement with plan. Emailed links for KellyMom and ABRW websites to pt. Will send report with protocol to Dr Smith, Dr. Jones.

Linda Lactation, IBCLC

Attachment G

Dialogue Essay for Abuse Screening

WORKING WITH ABUSED MOTHERS
by Cynthia Good Mojab, MS, IBCLC, RLC, CATSM

Everyone who works with new mothers - from IBCLCs and lay counselors to nurses and doctors - needs to be prepared to hear about abuse and needs to know what to do when they hear about it. Many women have histories of sexual abuse, physical abuse, rape, and/or domestic violence. This is not a rare situation. We need to know how to acknowledge what has been revealed, we need to be able to state the limits of our ability to respond to what has been revealed, and we need to be able to refer a mother to a source of support who is knowledgeable about both mental health and breastfeeding. Our ability to do this well will never be forgotten. If the healthcare provider is not a mental health professional, and depending on a great deal of context that would vary tremendously from situation to situation, the dialogue might look something like this:

> "Thank you for trusting me enough to share this with me. I imagine it was difficult for you to do so. I'm not an expert in this area, but I do know that many women have had experiences like yours and have struggled with infant feeding decisions because of those experiences. With a chance to talk with someone about what has happened in the past and what they are feeling now, many mothers have become comfortable with breastfeeding and have even found the breastfeeding experience healing and empowering. And, regardless of whether a mother breastfeeds directly, expresses her milk and feeds it to her baby, feeds her baby donor human milk, or formula feeds, talking with someone can help them move toward healing, which is important to the mother and her children. Here's the name and phone number of a counselor (or psychologist, psychiatrist, or therapist) I know. She specializes in women's issues like this and has a very good reputation in our community...."

There are a million ways to say all this. It could get changed with every verbal and nonverbal response a mother makes in the conversation, and there ought to be a great deal of listening done by the person saying it. But I hope it gives healthcare providers a general idea. The point is, saying something like this acknowledges what the mother has said, as well as gives her options she might not have known she had. It also requires the healthcare provider to track down, in advance, a mental healthcare provider who is knowledgeable about and supportive of breastfeeding. This may not be easy to accomplish.

I always address this issue up front whenever I teach pregnant couples about breastfeeding. I talk about how comfort with breastfeeding is more than physical -it's also emotional and social - how histories of abuse can impact breastfeeding, and how support is available to help mothers work toward healing and becoming more comfortable with breastfeeding. I've had women seek that support after class. It is very unlikely they would have done so without my first letting them know it was all right to do and that they were not alone in experiencing these kinds of challenges. The same mothers who are struggling with infant feeding decisions because of past abuse are also the ones who will struggle with mothering, although any mother can struggle with mothering due to the inherent difficulty of the maternal role. Abused mothers are at higher risk of developing postpartum depression and other mental health challenges. They need a ray of hope that help is available before they sink into despair.

© Cynthia Good Mojab, 2005. Used with Permission.

This text was first posted on June 28, 2005 to LACTNET, a netlist for professionals working in the field of breastfeeding and human lactation. It has been edited slightly here (CGM).

Chapter Eight

PUTTING IT TOGETHER

Applied Critical Thinking

Once the LC understands the individual elements of the history and assessment, the next task is blending these elements into a whole. Each part is not isolated, but rather linked by the critical thinking process. Critical thinking has many complex definitions, but is primarily the method of actively utilizing information to organize, observe, apply, question, examine, judge, and obtain additional facts to work through a process toward a conclusion (Potter & Perry, 2005). Critical thinking allows the LC to process in steps the identification of a problem (or multiple problems) and work toward resolution, most often a satisfied mother who determines the final outcome.

Below is a case study that illustrates how the LC can utilize information gathering techniques along with critical thinking skills through the natural flow of a consult. During this case, the baby was quiet on arrival which allowed for a conventional flow. If the baby had been fussy, the consultation would have started with a weight check, a rapid assessment, then straight into the feeding. The history review and interview would still be completed, just somewhat out of order. No element should be omitted because of organization of the form.

Details noted are not necessarily variations from the norm, but rather information triggers or red flags that indicate a need for additional exploration. As the LC reviews the history, she should ask questions as she is reading, rather than reading all the way through first, then asking questions. This will allow for a complete discussion.

Because this case study was written up after the fact and to allow for variations in practice methods, the critical thinking and questions are stated in generic terms. The intent is to give the reader a sense of the process. The setting was informal in the mother's home, and as a result, some of the elements of the interview deliberately create the perception of a casual conversation in order to help the mother relax. In addition, the questions are delivered using a variety of communication techniques, rather than the blunt statements below.

"Written" indicates statements on the history form completed by the mother.

"Critical Thinking" reflects the mental process of the LC in response to read, stated, or observed information.

"Question" is a verbal query by the LC in response to information intake and the critical thinking process.

"Observed" indicates found during assessment.

CASE PRESENTATION SIX-BABY J

Background

Setting is a home consultation by a PPLC. Referral initiated by Obstetrician. PPLC contacted by triage nurse; pt is having latch difficulties. When asked by the PPLC for additional details, nurse read from medical record, "Pt having latch difficulties, supply concerns. Refer to LC, consider Reglan if needed."

Critical Thinking: OB is pretty knowledgeable about basic BF issues, doesn't hesitate to refer to LC even for simple reassurance visits. OB and PPLC have good working relationship. Triage nurse is new to role, appears young and eager to support the pt. PPLC had not had much interaction with nurse and is unsure of experience or knowledge base.

Telephone contact by PPLC. Pt initially requesting intake assessment for supply concerns. When questioned about latch, states she also wants help weaning from nipple shield.

Critical Thinking: Pt is known to PPLC from prenatal classes; PPLC is reassured about baseline BF knowledge. First time mother.

History Form Review with Triggers

Written: Demographic-lives in downtown area. Ped is part of large group well known to PPLC.

Critical Thinking: Ped has traditionally been somewhat conservative with care recommendations, is well-liked by families, and seems to be very pt focused. Pt close to resources.

Question: How familiar are you with the resources in this area of town? How long have you lived here?

Written: Baby is 8 days old

Critical Thinking: Supply still being established, may be recovering from birth, should be starting to gain.

Written: Reason for Consult-difficulty latching, long feedings, slow weight gain

Critical Thinking: Latch problem coming up several times, probably primary focus. Haven't heard about long feedings-must get this defined. Also need to define slow weight gain since this may be expected based on infant history-we are only on day 8.

Question: Tell me why you need a lactation consult? Allow pt to verbally restate need for consult.

Written: Birth Wt-7.7lbs   D/C Wt 6.4lbs

Critical Thinking: What??? This would mean a weight loss of 16%.

Question: How many days were you and the baby in the hospital? How did you deliver? Were there complications?

Written: Other Wts.   Day 4-6.7lbs (13% loss, done at doctors office)   Day 5-6.10 lbs (with supplement) Started adding 1oz formula after breastfeeding, every feeding then used pumped milk for supplement.

Critical Thinking: This is pretty rapid growth for a kid who was so significantly depleted. Could the first weight be the result of human error?

Question: Did the hospital send home any discharge paperwork? What was the pediatrician's response to weight loss?

Written: Output in past 24 hours-7 bowel movements, bright yellow, moderate to large amount. Wet diapers-8

Critical Thinking: Seems like she is on track now.

Question: How many wet diapers did baby have in the past 24 hours? How many dirty diapers? Are you giving the baby anything in a bottle? If so, what?

Written: Most common infant state-sleepy.

Critical Thinking: Either real full or lethargic. I am betting full.

Question: How often is your baby in an active, alert state? How much time does your baby spend in a deep sleep? What does he (she) usually do after a feeding?

Written: Typical PP meds only; no medical issues.

Question: Are you taking any herbal remedies, any homeopathic remedies? If so, what? Are you taking a vitamin/mineral supplement? If so, is it one your doctor prescribed or one you purchased over-the counter? Are you taking anything else for health purposes?

Written: Delivered at 38.4 weeks by scheduled cesarean section for breech position. No complications.

Critical Thinking: Baby may be at near-term. Watch behaviors carefully, particularly organization and focus.

Question: How was this particular date chosen?

Written: Seen by LC twice; full feeding not observed.

Critical Thinking: LCs at this particular hospital have more patients than they can possibly handle. Sometimes tools are introduced early as a result.

Question: What did the LC observe and recommend?

Written: Supplement given in hospital by bottle for low weight.

Critical Thinking: Pt already using a nipple shield, bottle probably not going to make a huge difference at this point.

Question: How many times was infant supplemented? What was the rationale for bottle use? What was supplement?

Written: To nursery at night

Critical Thinking: Probably more bottles at night; nursery staff will over rather than underfeed. Why the excessive weight loss?

Question: Supplement verified above; when was baby back in room?

Written: Breastfeeding goals-written min of 6 months.
Critical Thinking: May be what she thinks I want to hear. Find out immediate goal.
Question: By the time I leave, what do you want to accomplish? How about in the next week? Month?

Written: Any other details that may be important? No
Critical Thinking: There is a lot missing here.
Question: Any incomplete elements, particularly with doctor's visits, feeding tools, the birth.

Most of the information from the mother's response was straightforward; however, she mentioned that even though she delivered by cesarean, the doctor had difficulty getting the baby out. "He was tucked up in the curve of the pelvic bone, which we even saw on ultrasound." This was not identified as a history trigger until the infant assessment.

Assessment with Triggers

Maternal Assessment

Observed: Bilateral scabbing, skin at nipple very pink. Wounds are at the base of the nipple, with an additional abrasion at the left tip.
Critical Thinking: Imprint of wound can indicate friction rubs at palate or from shield. Can also indicate clamping.
Question: Review signs of infection. How is mother currently treating wound? Is there any pain at rest? How have the wounds impacted feeding practices?

Observed: Shape of the nipple is well rounded; no variation
Critical thinking: If clamping, probably minimal duration. Will observe after feeding.
Question: Mother's self assessment after feeding regarding nipple tissue.

Infant Assessment

Observed: The infant was initially seen at rest, in a fairly deep sleep state. The facial asymmetry was observed immediately, leading to neck palpation where some contracture was felt at the left sternocleidomastoid muscle.

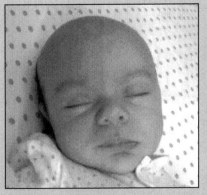

Baby J-before a feeding

This image shows Baby J asleep; it has been rotated for better viewing. According to his mother, he naturally turns his head to the right, very rarely to the left. His age is around 10 days.

- Note the droop at the left corner of his mouth, even with gravity pulling in the opposite direction.
- His nose is also slightly directed to the right.
- The crease below his chin is deeper at the left.
- In addition he has a suck callus or blister on his upper lip, and cracking from friction along the lower lip line, indicating that he is using both for stabilization.
- Eye height and size appears fairly balanced, as is head circumference.

The image below shows Baby J in a quiet alert state after a feeding.

- The suck callus, along with lower lip fissures, appear more pronounced, and both lips appear a little edematous.
- Even while awake with active muscle movement, the left side of the mouth is drawn.
- Chin creasing, as well as lower lip curve is more pronounced at the right.
- Baby J is leaning against a chair arm, but his head appears at midline, rather than tilted to the right with gravity.
- His left ear is lower than the right and appears flattened at the posterior.

Appears to have mild torticollis. Has not been medically diagnosed per mother.

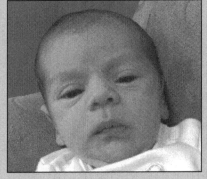

Baby J-After a feeding

Observed: Appears full term, developmentally appropriate.
Critical thinking: Organization may be better than anticipated from history.

Observed: Digital assessment revealed initial mild clamping.
Critical Thinking: No complications for the baby per pts history; consider suctioning or transition after c/section.
Question: Ask about deep suction, length of nursery stay, suctioning during hospitalization.

Feeding Assessment

Observed/Left Side: Attempted latch without shield. Infant will open wide with tongue extended, but unable to organize suck without rigid palate stimulation.
Critical Thinking: Mother will need tips for weaning from shield; identify actual feeding issues first.
Question: Have you tried feeding without the shield before now?

Observed: Shield loosely applied, infant "chewing" onto nipple.
Critical Thinking: Identifying point of trauma. Implement education.
Question: Questions will relate to education and return demonstration.

Observed: Breast assessment significant for rapid, forceful MER.
Critical Thinking: How is the baby handling this, is she clamping, slipping down?
Question: Does the feeding sensation change? Any pinching?

Observed/Right Side: Significant difficulties with latch at right side; multiple attempts.
Critical Thinking: Neck muscle variations appear to be creating positioning difficulties; utilize creative techniques.
Question: Questions will relate to education and return demonstration.

Observed: Intake of almost 4 ozs in 30 min.
Critical Thinking: Definite potential for oversupply, coupled with vigorous MER could lead to some signs of colic, reflux. Use anticipatory guidance.
Question: Confirm current feeding patterns.

Final Look

After the problem is identified and a plan created that is acceptable to the mother, baby, and support person, the LC should evaluate the consult. She will briefly scan the history and assessment to ensure that it is complete. She will then ask the mother to repeat back her recommendations for improvement, as well as determine if the mother or support person has questions or unmet needs, including making sure that the plan is acceptable to the mother. The evaluation has become a form of assessment at this point. She will conclude the consult with a statement of positive reinforcement.

If a follow up consult is needed, the LC will reinitiate the process. The physical and feeding assessment will be compared, another indication of the need for clear, definitive documentation.

The history taking will begin, again.

REFERENCES

American Academy of Pediatrics. Policy statement: the apgar score. Pediatrics. 2006; 117(4):1444-47.

Cadwell K, Turner-Maffei C, O'Connor B, Blair AC, Arnold L, Blair E. Maternal and infant assessment for breastfeeding and human lactation. Ed. 2. Sudbury: Jones and Bartlett; 2006.

Cotterman KJ. Reverse pressure softening: a simple tool to prepare areola for easier latching during engorgement. J Hum Lact. 2004; 20(2):227-37.

Cox JL, Holden JM, Sagovsky R. Detection of postnatal depression. Development of the 10-item Edinburgh Postnatal Depression Scale. Br J Psychiatry. 1987; 150:782-86.

Damato EG, Dowling DA, Standing TS, Schuster SD. Explanation for cessation of breastfeeding in mothers of twins. J Hum Lact. 2005; 21(3):296-304.

Declercq E, Sakala C, Corry M, Applebaum S. Listening to mothers II: report of the second national U.S. survey of women's childbearing experiences. J Perinat Educ. 2007; 16(4): 9-17.

Dunn S, Davies B, McCLeary L, Edwards N, Gaboury I. The relationship between vulnerability factors and breastfeeding outcomes. JOGNN. 2006; 35(1):87-97.

Gonzales K, et al. Evaluations of a lactation support service in a children's hospital neonatal intensive care unit. J Hum Lact. 2003; 19(3):286-92.

Hale, TW. Medications and mothers' milk. Ed 13. Amarillo, TX: Hale Publishing; 2008.

Humphries S. A nursing mothers herbal. Minneapolis: Fairview Press; 2003.

International Board of Lactation Consultant Examiners. Scope of practice guidelines. Adopted March 8, 2008. http://americas.iblce.org/home.php Accessed (Cited April 2008.)

Kassing D. Bottle feeding as a tool to reinforce breastfeeding. *J Hum Lact.* 2002: 18(1):56-60.

Language Line Services. http://www.languageline.com/. "Tips for Working with An Interpreter" (Cited April 2008.)

Lipson J, Dibble S., Minarek P. Culture and nursing care: a pocket guide. Ed.10. San Francisco: UCSF Nursing Press; 2002.

Lutz K. Abused pregnant women's interactions with health care providers during the childbearing year. JOGNN. 2005; 34(2):151-62.

Martin J. Is nipple piercing compatible with breastfeeding. J Hum Lact. 2004; 20(3):319-21.

Moody L, Slocumb E, Berg B, Jackson D. Electronic health records documentation in nursing: nurse's perceptions, attitudes and preferences. Comput Inform Nurs. 2004; 22(6):337-44.

Nommsen-Rivers L, Heinig J, Cohen R, Dewey K. Newborn wet and soiled diaper counts and timing of onset of lactation as indicators of breastfeeding inadequacy. J Hum Lact. 2008; 24(1):27-33.

Persing J, James H, Swanson J, Kattwinkel J. Prevention and management of positional skull deformities in infants. Pediatrics. 2003; 112(1):199-202.

Potter P, Perry A. Fundamentals of nursing. Ed. 6. St. Louis: Mosby; 2005.

Riordan J, Auerbach, K. Breastfeeding and Human Lactation. Third Edition. Sudbury: Jones and Bartlett; 2004

Smeltzer S, Bare B. Brunner and Suddarth's textbook of medical surgical nursing. Ed. 7. Philadephia: J. B. Lippencott. 1992.

Swartz M. Textbook of physical diagnosis: history and examination. Ed. 3. Philadelphia: W. B. Saunders Company; 1998.

ADDITIONAL RESOURCES

Books

Genna CW. *Supporting sucking skills in breastfeeding infants.* Sudbury: Jones and Bartlett; 2008.

Mohrbacher N, Stock J. *The breastfeeding answer book.* Ed. 3. Schaumberg: La Leche League International; 2003.

Smith L. *The lactation consultant in private practice: the ABC's of getting started.* Sudbury: Jones and Bartlett; 2003.

Walker M. *Core curriculum for lactation consultants.* Sudbury: Jones and Bartlett; 2002.

Journal Articles

Armstrong M, Caliendo C, Roberts AE. Pregnancy, lactation and nipple piercings. *AWHONN Lifelines.* 2006; 10(3):212-17.

Ayers J. The use of alternative therapies in the support of breastfeeding. *J Hum Lact.* 2000; 16 (1). 52-56.

Callahan S, Sejourne N, Denis A. Fatigue and breastfeeding: an inevitable partnership? *J Hum Lact.* 2006; 22 (2):182-87.

Cooke M, Sheehan A, Schmied V. A description of the relationship between breastfeeding experiences, breastfeeding satisfaction, and weaning in the first 3 months after birth. *J Hum Lact.* 2003; 19(2):145-56.

Damato EG, Dowling DA, Madigan EA, Thanattherakul C. Duration of breastfeeding for mothers of twins. *JOGNN.* 2005. 34(2). 201-9.

Hatton D, et al. Symptoms of postpartum depression and breastfeeding. *J Hum Lact.* 2005; 21(4):444-49.

Howie W, McMullen P. Breastfeeding problems following anesthetic administration. *J Perinatal Education.* 2006; 15(3):50-57.

Kim-Goodwin YS. Postpartum beliefs and practices among non-western cultures. *MCN.* 2003; 28(2):74-79.

Klingelhafer S. Sexual abuse and breastfeeding. *J Hum Lact.* 2007; 23(2):194-97.

Kumar S, Mooney R, Weiser L, Havstad S. The LATCH scoring system and prediction of breastfeeding duration. *J Hum Lact.* 2006; 22(4):391-96.

Leonard L. Breastfeeding higher order multiples: enhancing support during the postpartum hospitalization period. *J Hum Lact.* 2002; 18(4):386392.

Lewallen L, et al. Breastfeeding support and early cessation. *JOGNN.* 2006; 35(2):166-72.

List B, et al. Electronic health records in an outpatient breastfeeding medicine clinic. *J Hum Lact.* 2008; 24 (1):58-68.

Lutz K. Abused pregnant women's interactions with health care providers during the childbearing year. *JOGNN.* 2005; 34(2):151-62.

Martins P, Romphf L. Factors associated with newborn in-hospital weight loss: comparisons by feeding method, demographics and birthing procedures. *J Hum Lact.* 2007; 23(3):233-41.

Meier P. et al. A new scale for in-home test weighing for mothers of preterm and high risk infants. *J Hum Lact.* 1994; 10(3):163-68.

Radzyminski S. Neurobehavioral functioning and breastfeeding behavior in the newborn. *JOGNN.* 2004; 34(3):335-41.

Riordan J, Gill-Hopple K, Angeron J. Indicators of effective breastfeeding and estimates of breast milk intake. *J Hum Lact.* 2005; 21(4):406-12.

Roach J. Newborn stimulation: preventing over-stimulation is key for optimal growth and well-being. *AWHONN Lifelines.* 2004; 7(6):530-35.

Schlomer J, Kemmerer J, Twiss J. Evaluating the association of two breastfeeding assessment tool with breastfeeding problems and breastfeeding satisfaction. *J Hum Lact.* 1999; 15(1):35-38.

Smith L, Dayal V, Monga M. Prior knowledge of obstetric gestational age and possible bias of ballard score. *Obstet Gynecol.* 1999; 93:712-14.

Websites

Adoptive breastfeeding site created for mothers to offer general information, support, and encouragement. http://www.fourfriends.com/abrw/index.html. (Cited April 2008.)

Association of Professional Piercers; www.safepiercing.org. Professional organization website with a strong lay person focus intended for education and position statement purposes.

Diana West's site for mothers; www.lowmilksupply.org. Accessed for Shatavari article and survey. (Cited April 2008.)

Cynthia Good-Mojab's Lactational Psychology website, Lifecircle http://www.lifecirclecc.com/lactpsych.html and her family support site with articles at Ammawell, http://home.comcast.net/~ammawell/index.html. (Cited April 2008.)

Kelly Bonyata website primarily for mothers. www.kellymom.com. Accessed for "Oatmeal for Increasing Supply" and herbal galactagogues. (Cited April 2008.)

National Institute on Drug Abuse, www.nida.nih.gov/. Understanding Drug Abuse and Addiction; The Science of Addiction. (Cited April 2008.)

The New Ballard Score. Dr Jeanne Ballard's website dedicated to Newborn Gestational Assessment (homepage on the Internet). Available from: www.newbornmedicine.com. (Cited April 2008.)

The Newman-Goldfarb protocols for Induced Lactation, used for adopting mothers. Available from http://www.asklenore.info/index.html. (Cited April 2008.)

University of Michigan, Program for Multicultural Health. Enhancing Your Cultural Communication Skills, Cross-Cultural Interviewing Skills. Available from www.med.umich.edu/multicultural/ccp/questions.htm. (Cited April 2008.)

Yahoo internet tool site/search engine. Contains free language translation box. http://babelfish.yahoo.com/. (Cited April 2008.)

Other

International Lactation Consultants Association. Evidence-Based Guidelines for Breastfeeding Management during the First Fourteen Days. April 1999.

Personal communication, Veronia L. Ross MSN, RN/Information Systems Clinical Educator; dated April 14, 2008.

Personal communication, Chaka Davis RNC, MSN, MPH, IBCLC/Neonatal Outreach Educator for Midlands Perinatal Systems; dated April 23, 2008.

Personal communication/members of the Greater Columbia Area Mothers of Multiples Club; dated April 24-28.

COMMON ABBREVIATIONS LIST

Below is a list of abbreviations commonly used in the medical setting. In some instances, the same abbreviation is used with two different meanings. For example, ROM may mean range of motion to a physical therapist or in a long term care facility. However, in a birth center or in labor and delivery, ROM means rupture of membranes. For this monograph, abbreviations are intended for the mother-baby care setting.

a	before
AB, SAB	abortion, spontaneous abortion as in; miscarriage, pregnancy loss
Admit	admission (to healthcare facility)
All:	allergies
AM	morning
BCP	birth control pill
BM, bm	bowel movement
cc	milliliters, no longer approved, use ml
c/o	complains of
c/s	cesarean section
CST	cranio-sacral therapy
d/c	discontinued, can also mean discharged (from healthcare facility)
DOB	date of birth
drsg	dressing (refers to wound care)
EBM	expressed breast milk
EDC	estimated date of conception
f/u	follow up
grp	group
Gyn	gynecologist
hr, hrs	hour, hours
hx	history
ILC	inpatient lactation consultant
L, Lt	left
lb	pound
LC	lactation consultant
MD	physician

med	medication
mg	milligrams
ml	milliliter
MW	midwife
NBN	newborn
NICU	Neonatal Intensive Care Unit
nrsg	nursing, as in; care by a nurse
Nrsy	nursery
OB	obstetrician
OLC	outpatient lactation consultant
oz	ounces
pc	after
PCN	Penicillin
PCOS	polycystic ovarian syndrome
Ped	pediatrician
PICU	pediatric intensive care unit
PM	evening, night
PNV	prenatal vitamins
PPLC	private practice lactation consultant
prn	as needed
Pt	patient
qd	every day
q	every (as in: q2, every 2)
qfeed	every feeding
R, Rt	right
Rx	prescription, medication
s/s	signs and symptoms
sx	symptoms
tx	treatment, therapy
wks	weeks
wt	weight
y.o.	year old
x	for (as in: x8hours, for 8 hours)
$\bar{c}$	with
$\bar{s}$	without

INDEX

BIOGRAPHICAL INFORMATION

Denise Altman RN, IBCLC, LCCE

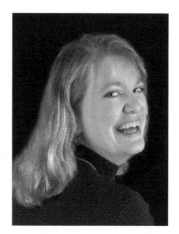

Denise Altman is a private practice lactation consultant and nurse educator. She currently owns and operates All The Best in Columbia, South Carolina. Prior to that, she worked in a variety of roles in the healthcare system from staff nurse to clinical educator.

Her business operates on a three tier system; prenatal education, lactation support, and professional resourcing. She is also a freelance writer and professional speaker. On a personal note, Denise is the mother of three children.

Made in the USA
Coppell, TX
15 January 2021

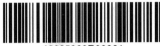